LOOKS THAT WORK

Also by Janet Wallach

Working Wardrobe

How to match your wardrobe to your professional profile and create the image that's right for you

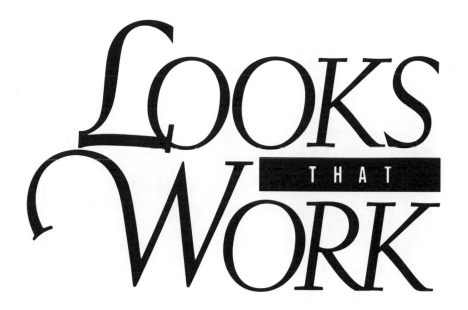

LOOKS THAT WORK

BY

JANET WALLACH

Illustrations by Martha Vaughan

VIKING

VIKING

Viking Penguin Inc., 40 West 23rd Street,
New York, New York 10010, U.S.A.
Penguin Books Ltd, Harmondsworth,
Middlesex, England
Penguin Books Australia Ltd, Ringwood,
Victoria, Australia
Penguin Books Canada Limited, 2801 John Street,
Markham, Ontario, Canada L3R 1B4
Penguin Books (N.Z.) Ltd, 182–190 Wairau Road,
Auckland 10, New Zealand

LIBRARY OF CONGRESS CATALOGING IN PUBLICATION DATA
Wallach, Janet, 1942–
   Looks that work.
   1. Clothing and dress.   2. Beauty, Personal.
I. Title.
TT507.W2169   1986   646'.34   85-41067
ISBN 0-670-80610-2

Printed in the United States of America

Produced for Viking by Ripinsky & Company
Designed by Laurel Vaughan
Composition, printing and binding by The Maple-Vail Book Manufacturing Group
Color printing by New England Book Components
The text of this book is composed in Garamond Light

To all the
women who struggle
to get dressed every day

Acknowledgments

With much appreciation to: Martha Vaughan for her dedication and talented art work; Laurel Vaughan for the design of the book; Neil Stuart for his creative cover concept; Amanda Vaill for her wise counsel and enthusiasm; Stacy Schiff for her patience and good humor; Harriet Ripinsky for her exuberance in seeing the project through; and Leona Schecter for her encouragement.

A special note of thanks to Hanne Merriman for her friendship and valued support, and to all of the women mentioned in the book who gave their valuable time and insights to this project.

Contents

Sending the Right Message

When Hatshepsut connivingly crowned herself Queen of Egypt during the 18th dynasty (ca. 1496–1468 B.C.), she realized very quickly that she had to dress the part: that was one way to establish her credibility. Like all those leaders before her (all those before her being men), she donned the traditional ceremonial costume worn for official portraits. This favorite fashion of the pharaohs consisted of a short skirt, a headcloth and a beard. Hatshepsut wanted to project the proper profile; she and her constituents knew what a leader was supposed to look like. Gender may not have mattered, but image did.

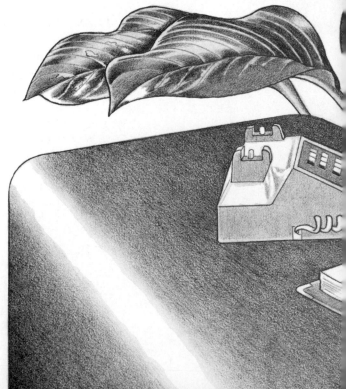

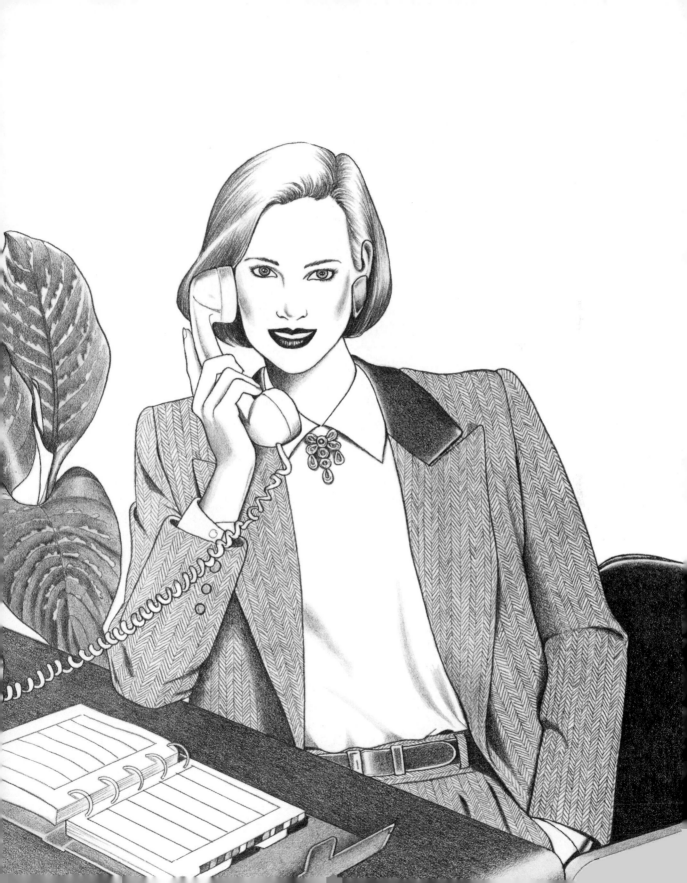

Some things have changed since then. Women can now achieve power without the dirty double-dealing that went on in Hatshepsut's day. Successful women don't dress in exactly the same clothes as their male peers. But, like Hatshepsut, many enterprising women have found out that it pays to project the right image. The problem is how to instill that image into a woman's clothing and appearance. There are no official costumes or uniforms that we can slip into. To complicate matters even further, different careers call for different images, and that requires different clothes. Deciding which outfit to wear is often a dilemma.

Up until fairly recently most women dressed by the rules of fashion. If the "right" hemline was above the knee, they wore their skirts above the knee. If the "right" color was red, they wore red. If the "right" look was broad shoulders or baggy pants, they wore those too.

But the rules of fashion have disappeared. There are no longer any "right" hemlines or hairstyles dictated by designers. Fashion is a free-for-all. However, a different set of rules has appeared; these are the rules of enterprise. For the woman of the 1980s, it is winning in her career, not winning the fashion game, that is important. The way we dress, and the image our clothes project, are more significant than ever before. To win the game, you have to play by the rules.

Simple enough, you might think. But, ah, there's a catch! The rules aren't the same for all the players. There are, in fact, three sets of rules—one for each of the three major career profiles. These profiles are the Corporate, the Communicator, and the Creative.

Almost any job of an enterprising woman, including volunteer work, falls into one of these three categories. By knowing which profile category you fit into and understanding how to dress for that profile, you can project the right image. You can easily follow the rules of the game and build an appropriate wardrobe for your career.

Think of a woman you know who is a banker, another who sells houses, and a third who is an artist. Should they dress alike? Of course not. It wouldn't suit their jobs and it probably wouldn't suit their personalities either. They may all want to look assertive, authoritative and professional, but each one has to do it in a way that's right for her. The banker, who fits the Corporate profile, needs a style that projects her efficiency and objectivity. The sales agent, who comes under the Communicator profile, should look sincere and friendly. The artist, who fits the Creative profile, wants to emphasize her imagination and innovation.

CLOTHES SEND YOUR MESSAGE

Looks That Work is about how clothes communicate your message. All too often we feel controlled by our clothes rather than the other way around. Clothing is a tool, and by planning a wardrobe strategy, you can make your clothes work effectively for you. You can get your clothes to say what you want them to say about you. When it comes to dressing, the choices that women have are almost endless, so it's easy to see why so many women dress in ways that send out mixed signals. This book will help you find your career profile and show you what kinds of clothes are appropriate for it. It will teach you how to build an effective, flexible wardrobe that will help you look and feel attractive, yet express your message as a professional. This is truly a working wardrobe.

I spent twenty years in the fashion industry, first as a sportswear designer, and then as fashion merchandising director of Garfinckel's, a large specialty store chain. In both of these positions I attended meetings and conferences with store executives and other professional people in the fashion industry. I dressed in a way that was businesslike yet I hoped showed imagination and fashion innovation. My working profile was Creative. When I began writing my first book, *Working Wardrobe,* I left Garfinckel's and set up an office in the basement of my house. My working wardrobe became a sweatshirt and jeans, and I was happy to be wearing that. My working profile was still Creative. However, I was no longer dressing for image but for comfort. My clothing had gone from designer labels to Levis, and I was comfortable in each at the appropriate time. The wardrobe that works for you depends on the work you do.

After the book was finished I was asked to make an author's tour around the United States. This involved television talk shows, radio programs and newspaper interviews as well as fashion seminars at leading department stores. The first question I asked myself was, "What am I going to wear?" Now this may sound odd coming from the author of a primer on dressing. But the truth is, I wasn't sure what I wanted to say about myself and I knew that the way I looked would be the key to being a good Communicator. I realized that the moment I stepped in front of a television camera, one reporter or a roomful of working women, a judgment would be made about my credibility. I wanted to look professional and appropriate. I had to be sure that I projected the image of authority, that I understood fashion and also understood the needs of professional businesswomen. The audiences were mostly career women or women who wanted to begin a career, so I had to project credibility as a person who understood their problems in terms of work and dressing. I felt it was important that the audience could identify with the way I looked. But I also had to look like the woman I was: a woman who had spent twenty years in the fashion business.

In going through this process, I realized that I wouldn't be viewed in a Creative role, but rather in the role of a Communicator. I had to tell the audience about my background and make them feel that I understood their needs. No longer working alone in comfort in the basement of my house, I would have high visibility, appearing before large numbers of people.

Many women are not used to this sort of high visibility. They may want it because they realize it can help them achieve their career goals faster and possibly more smoothly, but they may also feel uncomfortable with it, even afraid. Because with that visibility go many responsibilities; most importantly, looking and acting in a way that appropriately represents their position. As one executive search consultant told me, she was frustrated by women who wanted front office jobs but looked as though they belonged in the *back* office.

In my mother's generation, and to some extent even in mine, women stayed home and raised children and had visibility only when they achieved some recognition doing volunteer work, such as PTA or church or community fund-raising. My mother, for example, was quite active as an officer in one charitable organization. Once a year her group had a special luncheon in honor of its most productive workers. My mother was asked to sit on the dais, which was a privileged and highly visible position. Although she was not particularly interested in clothes, I distinctly remember long and numerous telephone calls between my mother and her friends about what to wear to the luncheon. This was the one time a year when she would be seen in an authoritative role. This was her moment of visibility and she wanted to dress the part.

All of that is quite different now for the more than half of all women who work. A good number of us are seen very often, more often indeed than some of us would like. Judgments are made about us constantly. Like it or not, fair or unfair, we are all judged by our appearance.

Probably the most difficult part of visibility is deciding how you want to be perceived. To figure this out you might ask yourself several questions: How do I *like* to dress? What is the image of my organization? How do others in my organization dress? Who is the audience I am addressing?

In the book *Upward Mobility,* edited by Catalyst, a women's non-profit career guidance organization, the writers say, "Your boss and co-workers form a certain opinion of you, and because of that conception, they consequently expect you to behave, dress, and perform in a certain way. Eventually, their conception of your image can become a self-fulfilling prophecy. Maybe you were denied that supervisor's job because you dress more like a secretary than an ambitious, talented career woman . . . Superficial matters like dress and speech do matter in the business world. Certainly competence is more important, but substance without appropriate style and behavior won't get you very far."

These words suggest that there *is* an appropriate, professional way to dress. Certainly these words crop up over and over again in anything relating to career dressing. They seem easy to define at first, but actually the definitions change with every situation. What is appropriate for a financial manager may be absurd for a fine artist. What is professional in one office may be all wrong in another.

This ties in, too, with the matter of that overworked expression dressing for success. The question is, success in what? The practice of imitating men's dress to give an impression of success has been discarded by a majority of women. In the conservative, corporate world, dressing for success may be a matter of choosing what kinds of women's clothing best express your business style in the same ways that men's clothing does for them. As a television news anchorwoman, real estate saleswoman, art director or newspaper journalist, however, you need to look at different symbols and apply them to your wardrobe.

COSTUMES AND ROLES. Obviously there is no one costume that will apply across the board. There are too many kinds of roles and too many requirements for those roles. But the right costume for a given role gives you an aura of appropriateness. It gives you the confidence to perform the part well. Not only does the costume identify you for the audience, but it helps reinforce your own feelings about your role.

My young son, Michael, is a good example. When Michael was about five years old, one of his favorite games was Superman. He would get all dressed up in trousers, a long sleeve shirt and a jacket. Then he would announce himself proudly: "Hi, Mommy, I'm Clark Kent." "Hello, Clark," I would answer, glad to go along with the game. Within seconds he would stop me and say, "Uh oh, somebody's in trouble. I better get Superman." With that, he would dash off to the corner of the room, slip off his trousers, his shirt and his pants. Lo and behold, underneath he had on red shorts and a blue T-shirt with the big red and yellow "S." He was wearing the costume of Superman. Now he could perform Herculean feats: He was dressed for the part.

LOOK THE PART. You don't have to play Superman (or Lois Lane) to realize that the right clothes make a difference. They help you feel better qualified for the job. If you are at a place of business, you're much more likely to feel businesslike in a suit and blouse than in a sweatshirt and jeans. On the other hand, you'll have more fun on the weekend if you wear casual clothes.

Not too long ago, I moderated a fashion show in Knoxville. Most of the models were dressed in suits. But one model wore a soft, flowing skirt and loose jersey top. "I feel like I'm on the beach in Venice, California," she said. There's no doubt that our clothes help set our mood.

At the same time, a lot of people feel more comfortable when they are dressed like the rest of the group. Almost every one of us has been in a situation where we are dressed one way and everyone else another. It might be at a party where you have on your fanciest dress and the other women are all in jeans, or it could be a first day at the office with you in pants and all the other women wearing dresses.

Whatever the reason—whether it is wearing clothes that are decidedly different from everyone else's, or wearing clothes that are uncomfortable because of fit, style or fabric—the wrong clothes make us feel awkward and out of place. I remember going to a meeting with a run in my pantyhose. All I could think about was hiding my leg so no one would see the run. Women executives at all levels of management are affected by their clothes. That's why it's important to have a clear-cut strategy for wardrobe planning.

Most of us have also had the pleasure of wearing something that we feel makes us look attractive. That gives us confidence, and the confidence helps us to do a good job. All of these positive feelings become self-fulfilling. The better we feel about ourselves, the better the job we do. Much of this self-confidence comes from knowing we are dressed appropriately.

One of the most effective ways that women can establish their place in their field is to dress professionally and look their part. Unfortunately, this does not always happen. Look around an office and you will see the men dressed in a certain identifiable manner. Look at the women and you will probably see a wide variety of styles.

Although women are moving in the direction of professional dressing, there is still an incredible gap between what we want to project and what we actually say with our appearance. Many women are sending the wrong message. If they have adopted the business suit, they may not have adapted it to their own personalities. All too often the cut or fabric is boring, too severe or too threatening. And women who have taken a softer approach in their dressing may be sending out a message that is too casual or too sexual.

There is a way to make your appearance businesslike yet feminine. There is plenty of room for attractive dressing in the working world, but it must be modified by certain guidelines. The guidelines are suggested by your personality, the function of your job, the image of your organization, and the audience you are addressing. Each of you can achieve a look that is professional yet feminine, competent yet soft. Dressing appropriately can help you move effectively in your career. Dressing inappropriately can have the opposite result.

Even as women have gained jobs and visibility in traditionally male-dominated areas, their salaries still fall considerably below their male counterparts'. A great deal of this discrepancy has been due, without doubt, to a pre-established bias against women. One of the most effective ways we can communicate our ability and our seriousness is by dressing appropriately. But all too often we aren't sure what we want to say with our wardrobes or how we should say it. This book will show you how to send the right message. One of the easiest ways to signal your professionalism is to have your clothes speak for you.

THE PSYCHOLOGY OF DRESSING: YOU ARE WHAT YOU WEAR

Clothes talk. They say volumes about how we feel, how we want to be perceived, how we see others. We communicate through our appearance. The way we package ourselves sends out a particular message.

Major marketing corporations spend millions of dollars annually deciding how to package their products. The difference between a product that has been packaged well and one that hasn't may be the difference between success and failure. No one will know if the cookies taste good if they never buy the box. And one package won't work for everything. You wouldn't expect to buy chocolate chip cookies wrapped in a pale blue box from Tiffany's. The box looks pretty, but it doesn't give enough information to make us want to buy the product. Each package should say something special about the contents and each product must be packaged appropriately for its audience.

The same applies to people. You may have more talent than anyone else in your field, but unless you present the right kind of package, no one will bother to find out about you. You may get passed over for promotions or never even hired in the first place if your appearance is not right.

The tricky part is to know what *is* appropriate. It really is fairly easy to find out once you clearly understand your feelings about yourself, your job function, your organization and your audience.

SIGNALING YOUR FEELINGS. Successful women generally look successful. They wear clothes that look attractive on them, are well-groomed, speak well and posture themselves with confidence. The message that comes across is that they feel good about themselves—and you probably feel good about them too. Just remember: They didn't start out successful—they became that way.

But we don't all have such positive feelings about ourselves. We may all want to get ahead but our self-doubts inhibit us. These negative feelings come through in the way we dress and, unfortunately, our appearance may shout that same negative message.

Very often negative feelings come from being unsure about the way you look. If you feel confident that your clothes, hairstyle and makeup all help you look attractive, you will communicate that message to your audience. On the other hand, if you have doubts about your appearance, those feelings will also come through. As quiet and unassuming as you may *want* to be, the message will be loud and clear.

If you feel negative about yourself, if you look in the mirror and want to cringe, it is time to rethink the way you dress.

The place to begin is with your own picture of yourself. If you don't like what you see, others may not either. The real picture may not be so bad, but your negative feelings will color and distort it. Your posture won't be as good, your voice as strong, and your whole self will telegraph a lack of confidence. If you don't have confidence in yourself, why should anyone else?

There are some women who deliberately dress in a way that makes them unattractive. They believe that an attractive appearance takes away from their credibility; it is seen as a sign of self-indulgence or frivolity. These women feel that in order to be taken seriously, they must show no interest in the way they look. But in reality almost everyone, male or female, cares about his or her appearance. By presenting an unattractive picture, you are saying that you don't care about yourself or care enough about your audience to make yourself more attractive.

Other women present an unattractive appearance because they feel guilty about their careers. They may have struggled for years to do better than their mothers, to have more interesting lives and more rewarding experiences. Yet as hard as they have worked for their own advancement, they can't let themselves enjoy the pleasure of being attractive.

Says California psychologist Beth Milwid, "Understand that you may be getting more than your mother did. Work on how guilty that makes you feel . . . you are going to get more than your mother. Don't undo your own possibilities by dressing like a dump because you're guilty getting more than your mother. Remember, your mother wants to make peace with you before she dies. It's everything in your mother's self-interest to have you looking wonderful. It's everything in your mother's self-interest to have you doing great. Don't worry about outdoing her. Time to make peace."

Some women make themselves unattractive out of anger, i.e. anger about being a woman. They feel shortchanged. But the more unattractive they look, the more they will suffer.

Millie Kondracke, a Washington, D.C. psychiatric social worker, says of these women, "They get pleasure out of looking like the underdog. If you give a message to the world that 'I don't care about myself, don't care about how I look,' why should anybody else care?"

There are women who feel so unattractive—out of guilt or anger, or for other reasons—that they use their clothing as a hiding place. Kondracke often works with women who feel this way. She says, "As they start to feel they have the right to be feminine, to be a woman, you will see that their clothes start to change. As they feel they have the right to compete with other women, and that they can compete successfully—competition being a good thing, not a bad thing—that they have the right to be noticed, they don't have to hide. As they start to feel better about themselves . . . you notice a change in their appearance. You notice they want to change their hairstyle, they want to buy some new clothes. They feel they have the right to be attractive."

There are also women who are afraid that being attractive is threatening to the men around them. Says Kondracke, "Women argue that if we're very attractive they won't hire us, they won't think we're smart, they won't listen to us. The men I talk to say it's not true . . . I do think that being attractive, dressing attractively, not masculine, is something that women should strive for."

The imitation man's look—the woman in the menswear tailored navy blue suit, white shirt and bow tie—has become prevalent around the country. Kondracke says, "The picture they're trying to present is that 'I am masculine, I can handle this as well as any man and I can be as masculine or as manly or as powerful' or whatever they think men are—that there's something wrong about the appeal of sexuality." She believes these women are saying that there's something wrong with being a woman. But Kondracke adds, "I don't know why we should want to be like men."

As women we have both a right and an obligation to ourselves to look attractive, especially if we want to advance in our careers. The important thing to remember is to match that attractiveness with what is appropriate for our position.

But most of us don't have such a clear picture in our heads. Instead, our self-image is unfocused or distorted. We have to learn how to put ourselves in a successful career picture.

VISUALIZING SUCCESS. One way to develop a positive picture of yourself is through the process of visualization. If you can see a picture of yourself that you like, one that says, "I'm terrific. I can get the job done. I can do even bigger and better things," then you are on the right track. By visualizing success you can learn to do two things: To plan out your career and to present yourself attractively.

Cindy Ryan is a highly successful attorney in Los Angeles. But her profession has not always been law. She had been a professional tennis player, and she has since applied the strategy she learned then to her legal career.

Ryan says, "I'd been a tennis player on the circuit, and you learn to visualize your situation and act accordingly. Because in tennis, basically, you have to assess the audience or the opponent—however you want to characterize it—and make some decisions about how you're going to influence the game. So, I made a game plan for myself."

Before a match Ryan would watch her opponent play and size up her abilities. After a few games, she says, "I would tend to visualize how the other played. I could see her on the court. I could see her strengths and weaknesses. Then I would see myself on the court. I would see my strengths and weaknesses. Then we'd play the match—mentally. I would literally visualize how the match would go. The better I was at visualizing twenty-four hours in advance of the game, the more likely I was going to win. The times that I didn't do this were often the times that I lost. If I could play the match out in my head, often times I literally would perform almost in an identical fashion.

"It's sort of like your mind has a tremendous power. You gain confidence because you've played the match once before. I think that's partly what's happening with clothing too."

The more you practice visualizing yourself in a courtroom, in the boardroom, appearing on television, making a presentation, or closing a sale, the more successful you will be. Similarly, the better you visualize yourself as appropriately, professionally and attractively dressed, the easier it will be to actually look that way.

To help visualize yourself in your role, look at the picture carefully. Set the surroundings: an office, a conference room, an auditorium. Look at the other people who are there. Look at your audience, whether they are colleagues or clients. Carefully observe how they are dressed. Does your appearance fit in with the picture? How do you compare with other people in your position in your organization? In your field? How does your image compare with the image of your organization? Do you dress in a high-fashion style while your company is conservative? Do you dress in pants but all the other women wear skirts? Put the leaders of your organization in the picture. Do you look like a member of their team? Put yourself at a conference table. Do you look as though you belong there?

Now picture yourself making a presentation. Are people paying attention to what you say, or is your appearance too distracting? Are they listening to you or are they staring at your hairstyle or your dress? Change the picture: You are closing a sale with some important clients. Look at the people you are doing business with. Then look at yourself. Do you look enough like them so that they feel you are on their side? Or do you look threatening, like an opponent? Then put yourself in front of a large audience. Do people look at you or are you so bland they find other things to do while you are speaking? Are you distracting them with your jingling bracelet or your dangling earrings? What can you do to improve each of these pictures?

If you still are not sure how you should look, or how you want to look, go through the pages of magazines such as *Savvy, Self, Working Woman, Glamour, Vogue* or *Harper's Bazaar.* You will see dozens of different looks and styles. Try them out in your mind. See which ones fit with your picture of yourself. Some will look ridiculous. Others may work but will need some slight adjustment. Others may suit you exactly.

In order to visualize yourself appropriately you need to know the image of your organization and your field. The authors of *Upwardly Mobile* say, "Most companies have an image and would like their employees to conform to it. There is also a distinct image or business style that accompanies every profession. A lawyer, for example, is expected to dress and carry herself one way, while a publicity agent is expected to look and act quite different."

FINDING A JOB TO FIT YOUR PERSONALITY. It is always important to realize that your own personality should be in tune with your job. Naturally, the ideal position is one in which you feel entirely comfortable; one in which your personality fits in with the personality of your organization. If you are a creative person, you will undoubtedly be happiest in a job that demands your creativity and in an organization that appreciates it. If you enjoy letting your imagination run free, then being an accountant may be too restrictive for your needs while working in an advertising agency may be just right. If you are a person who enjoys meeting new people, you probably shouldn't be cooped up in a research laboratory but out selling the company's products.

When you are organizing your wardrobe, be aware of the organization and the field you are in. Jean Sisco, a management consultant and a director on the boards of eight major corporations says, "The first thing I would do is to take a good look at and understand what my job entailed; where my contacts would be; what type of work I would be doing most of the time; what do I need for work comfort. Then, I think you look at what the lead women, the top level women in that organization wear. What do your competitors outside the organization wear. Then, I would turn to what I find to be my style, the thing that I feel best in, look best in, and adapt that within the general framework. So that you are yourself, you feel you look well, and you aren't going to be blatantly upstaging anyone."

According to the authors of *Upwardly Mobile,* "Having a personality clash with your job can lead to job dissatisfaction and confusion regarding career choice. Perhaps you think you hate accounting, but what you really might hate is dressing conservatively and adhering to a strict nine-to-five routine."

If you are considering joining a new organization or if you are unhappy where you are now, take a look around you. If you do not feel comfortable with the way people look, you may be in the wrong place. Think of yourself as an actress in a play. If everyone is dressed by one costume designer, *you* don't want to be dressed by someone else. If you are, you won't look part of the cast—you'll look as if you belong in a different production and the audience will not respond to you.

One young woman I talked to had just such an experience. Ellen had graduated from law school and joined a small law firm. She enjoyed dressing in a variety of suits and dresses with bright scarves or other accessories while the other women in the firm always wore navy or gray suits and little foulard ties. "I was very clothing conscious, appearance conscious and I didn't want to be somebody else," she says. The clothing was symbolic of a mismatch. "What I wanted to say to the firm was that if they didn't like me on my terms, we were a bad match. We were a terrible match, horrible. I discovered after a time that I didn't want to be there. I'm sure that some of the men in the firm felt uncomfortable with me because I wasn't playing it their way." Ellen has since joined an organization where there is room for her personality to come through in her clothes as well as in her work. She is much happier and far more productive.

When you are interviewing for a job, look carefully at the other people in the firm and how they dress. You will learn a great deal about the organization. Judy Mapes is an executive recruiter with an international placement firm. She says, "I think women should observe the culture of where they work and dress accordingly. If they're not comfortable in that kind of dress, then they're in the wrong culture and they ought to do something else. People ought to be where they're comfortable, and that includes work. If they find that the culture is anathema to the way they feel, they're in the wrong job. Then they're going to complain that they don't get ahead because they're women. In fact, they're in the wrong place and none of it works. It should all feel right. You should recognize yourself in other employees: the way they dress, act, talk, feel, where they live, what they do, and what their interests are. It should all fit, or it should be where you want to be—maybe not where you are, but where you see yourself going, or the next step."

You should also be aware of other reasons why you may have chosen a particular field. It is up to you, of course, to decide if your choice is a good one or if it is inappropriate to your personality.

Says Beth Milwid, "We all go into our industries for unconscious reasons. There's something in our past we're working through. Whether it's a wonderful thing that we were given as a child from a parent that we dearly love and want to continue—a lot of people who were well-educated go into education—or maybe it was a trauma that we went through and unconsciously we have picked a way to work it out. . . . We all do it. You need to know why you're in your business. You need to connect with it as you work. You need to be proud of it. You can do this in your dress."

Once you have chosen your field, it is important to be aware of the way others in it present themselves. This is the way that people in the industry communicate with each other. It is their private language. If you want to be a part of that community, you must speak the same language.

Milwid explains: "Every industry has its culture. You need to understand the culture of the industry, unconsciously where it's coming from, and where you're coming from if you want to be in it. Make it conscious and then understand the rules of the game." Remember, too, that your audience has certain expectations. We expect the person who sells Rolls Royces to dress differently from the person selling Fords. We want our bankers to look like bankers, our artists to look like artists. It gives us confidence that they can do the job.

Know Yourself

Take this quiz to find out which profile suits you best.

1. Do you visualize yourself:

a) Behind a desk in a large corporation ☐
b) Persuading a jury in a courtroom ☐
c) Teaching in a classroom ☐
d) Anchoring a television news program ☐
e) Doing publicity for a cosmetics firm ☐
f) Designing clothes for a fashion firm ☐

2. You would like a career such as:

a) Sandra Day O'Connor/ Supreme Court Justice ☐
b) Nancy Kassebaum/Senator ☐
c) Mary Wells Lawrence/ Head of an ad agency ☐
d) Jane Pauley/Television personality ☐
e) Meryl Streep/Actress ☐
f) Donna Karan/Fashion designer ☐

3. Would you rather:

a) Read a legal contract ☐
b) Balance a checkbook ☐
c) Investigate a story ☐
d) Sell someone something ☐
e) Talk to artists ☐
f) Invent a recipe ☐

4. Do you like to wear:

a) A traditional suit every day ☐
b) A dark dress and jacket every day ☐
c) Suits and dresses with a little flair ☐
d) Skirts and sweaters, interesting jewelry ☐
e) The latest fashion ☐
f) Clothing as outrageous as possible ☐

5. Your favorite magazine is:

a) *Fortune* ☐
b) *Forbes* ☐
c) *People* ☐
d) *Glamour* ☐
e) *Vanity Fair* ☐
f) *Vogue* ☐

6. Do you enjoy:

a) Managing a team ☐
b) Playing on a team ☐
c) Cheerleading for a team ☐
d) Reporting about a team ☐
e) Writing a team song ☐
f) Leading a team band ☐

7. Do you like to dress:

a) Like most of your colleagues ☐
b) The same way every day ☐
c) A little different from your colleagues ☐
d) With some interesting touches ☐
e) In the latest fashion ☐
f) As outrageously as possible ☐

8. Do you view dressing for work as:

a) A career tool ☐
b) Simply a necessity ☐
c) Mildly interesting ☐
d) Sometimes fun ☐
e) A way to express yourself ☐
f) An art form ☐

9. Do others see you as:

a) Efficient--you get the job done ☐
b) Competent--a good manager ☐
c) Friendly--you like to be with people ☐
d) Sincere--they'd buy anything from you ☐
e) Original--you're always different ☐
f) Inventive--you always have new ideas ☐

10. Your favorite acting role would be:

a) Faye Dunaway/*Network* ☐
b) Joan Collins/*Dynasty* ☐
c) Lauren Bacall/*Woman of the Year* ☐
d) Sally Field/*Absence of Malice* ☐
e) Jane Fonda/*Julia* ☐
f) Diane Keaton/ *Annie Hall* ☐

EVALUATION: *If you answered mostly "a" or "b" you prefer the Corporate profile; mostly "c" or "d" you are a Communicator; mostly "e" or "f" you are a Creative profile.*

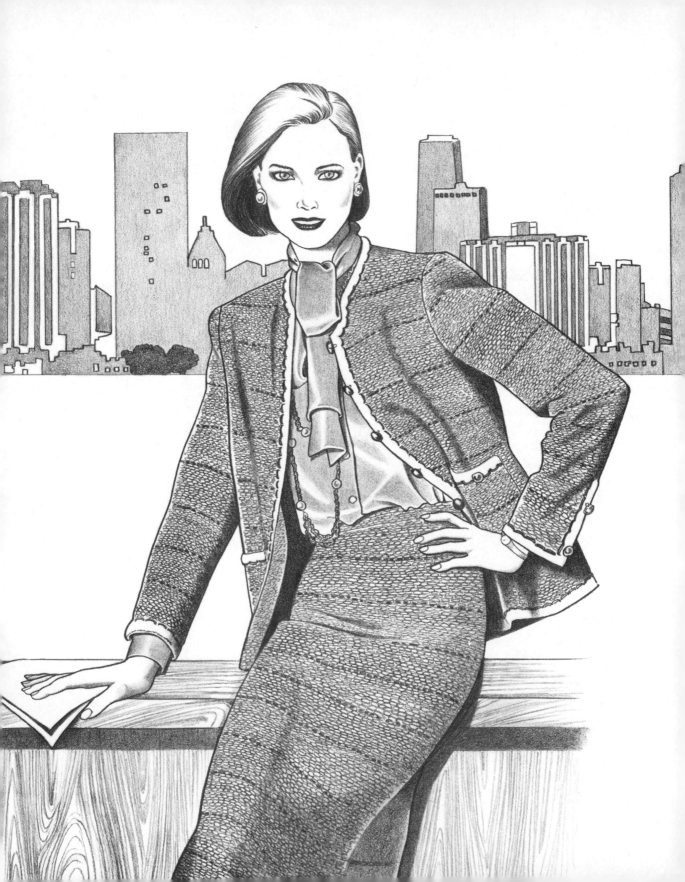

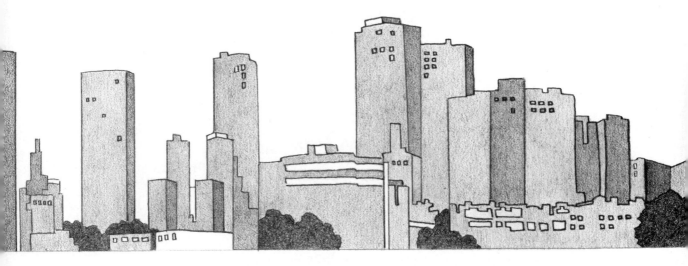

C H A P T E R   I I

The Corporate Profile

Although there are a wide variety of career opportunities open to women, almost all of them fall into one of three profiles: Corporate; Communicator; and Creative. Each area is distinctly different and marked by its own identity. However, the definitions are broad and there is plenty of room within each profile to express your individual personality. You may not see every type of job listed here but can apply the factors to your position to see where it fits.

THE CORPORATE PROFILE   31

Women have traditionally taken a very narrow definition of successful dressing for the work world and assumed that a mannish navy or gray flannel suit was the only route to follow. But as women are more and more accepted in the work force, we are learning that professional dressing does not exclude attractive, feminine looks.

THERE IS ROOM FOR YOUR PERSONALITY

While you are considering your career profile, it is important to take your own personality into account. You may prefer dressmaker details to menswear tailoring, dark colors to bright ones, or silks and suedes to tweeds and gabardine. There is room in each profile for your personal preferences and your style. For example, you may be a bank executive who enjoys wearing Chanel suits. While it is true that they are not the traditional tailored look that is associated with this Corporate profile, they are classic, constructed suits that give you an efficient and self-confident appearance.

There are times when you may want to incorporate looks from more than one profile. For instance, you may typically fit the Creative profile but on occasion want to relate more to the corporate world. A designer who needs financial backing may want to look more conservative when approaching her banker. Or, a lawyer whose client is in the fashion business may want to appear more innovative for those meetings.

Travel and leisure time also allow for more experimentation. There is information in every profile that can help you in your career profile and in your "off-the-job" life.

You may find that although you understand your own job needs, you are not so sure of your company's image. It may very well be that that image is somewhat fuzzy and not well defined. In fact, many firms are now hiring consultants to sharpen their image and train employees to conform their work and dress to the new look. The idea is to form more of a unified organization. IBM set the trend when it developed a dress code to stress its business image. The company's salesmen and executives were expected to wear dark suits and white shirts. This uniformity suggested that the entire corporation had a unified professional attitude. One nationwide real estate firm now asks its sales representatives to wear a bright gold blazer. This jacket immediately identifies members of that company and, at the same time, establishes a friendly yet professional attitude for the agents and the firm. Some organizations want a strict business look, others are more laid-back. When in doubt, watch how the highest ranking woman in the firm dresses.

Be aware of what the company is trying to say. You may find that this fits right in with your thinking, or you may be uncomfortable with it. If you are not happy with the company's image, ask yourself why. It may be that you are uncomfortable because it means making a change in your own appearance. But consider all of the aspects of that change. I asked one young woman who worked for a very conservative, male-oriented company if she resented her Corporate profile. "Not at all," she said. "It's very easy. You can have your freedom on the weekends." If, however, you find that the company image goes against your personality, you may need to make more than a change in clothes. You may want to make a career change, either by changing jobs within your organization, moving to a different company, or even changing fields.

Three factors go into the definition of a career profile. These are a) the job function itself; b) the particular organization and its image; and c) the broader look at the field or industry.

The Corporate profile includes administrative and line functions in urban companies in the fields of finance, law, consumer products and heavy industry. There is an emphasis on factual detail and advancement comes through upward reach (climbing the corporate ladder). The audience is composed of peers at the same professional level. These areas have been traditionally male-oriented and conservative in tone. For men and women in these fields, appearance is still conservative; that is, constructed suits and tailored dresses, solid colors or subtle patterns, and simple accessories.

The job functions that fall under the corporate umbrella range from accountant to attorney to administrator, as well as line responsibilities such as budgeting, production, personnel management and running a division. Some of the industries that are included are accounting, banking, brokerage, insurance, law, government and manufacturing.

TEAM PLAY. In all of these areas there is a major emphasis on teamwork. Belonging to a team is an important aspect, even a motivating factor for the Corporate person. The personality of the team becomes fused with the personality of the Corporate player. There is a strong sense of teamwork, teammates, and even team uniform. In law firms that specialize in major corporate work or that have high-profile clients, the partners generally wear well-cut clothes and look as successful as their clients. Trial attorney F. Lee Bailey is often seen in very expensive suits, for example. Conversely, lawyers who represent the public interest tend to dress down, like consumer advocate Ralph Nader, who is sometimes seen wearing rumpled suits. Other members of their firms are expected to dress like Bailey or Nader. Those people who fit in with the team, and are happy to be part of the team, are the ones who will succeed. Those who feel threatened by it or resent it or are threatening to it generally will not last long.

It is important for women to remember that the rules of the game were established a long time ago, and that they were set by men. Men have always been willing to play by these rules; otherwise they didn't hang around very long. Nonconformists left (and still leave) to form their own firms or to go into different fields. A woman will be accepted on the team far more easily if she plays by the same rules rather than trying to change them. The rules were made to reward those who are part of the team; they were not made to ostracize women.

People who gain acceptance and climb the corporate ladder play the team way. These people may show leadership, and to some degree initiative and independence, but it is generally of a non-threatening nature. It is done in an acceptable, appropriate way. Their career growth comes, after all, from within the organization. The team's managers decide who gets ahead and how fast. They watch to see how well a person functions within the framework of the organization. It is this upward reach that is one of the distinguishing elements of the Corporate profile. Because judgments about your growth come from above, being perceived as a team player is one of the most critical factors for your success.

The fastest and easiest way to identify yourself as a member of a team is to wear the team uniform. The man's business suit or "uniform" evolved over a century of time. It is an easy way to dress, requires few decisions, appears unfussy and thus allows both the wearer and the audience to concentrate on the essentials. Even though it is a uniform, there is still room for personal expression. The color, the fabric and the cut, plus the choice of accessories, all allow for individuality.

Wearing the uniform immediately says that you want to be on the team and are ready, willing and able to play by the rules of the team for the gain of the overall team.

This may be a difficult concept for some women to accept. We were not generally brought up to be team players but rather to be the team's mascots or cheerleaders; to cheer for the team but to do it with our backs to the players. In many cases we did not know or care what the rules were or how the players play the game. They were our team, but only from the sidelines. Similarly in the corporate world, we have been the supporting cast. Learning to be full members of the team is one of the biggest challenges women are facing.

Many women have the ability and the desire to be on the team, but don't understand the rules and dislike wearing the uniform, something we, as women, have not been required to do. The uniform is as much, if not more, a part of the team as any other single element. Men, in fact, are often quite proud of their particular uniform. For them, their school or club tie confirms that they are members of an elite group. Women traditionally have had a somewhat opposite view of dressing. A woman who walks into a room and sees someone else in her same outfit is sure to cringe. Yet there are some women who take refuge in seeing others dressed identically to them.

Judy Mapes, for example, told me she went to an all-girls school and that she never resented wearing a uniform because it represented one of the best schools in her city. She was proud to be seen in the uniform and identified as a member of that team. When she was older and joined a business firm, she immediately adapted the team uniform. Once again, she was proud to identify with that organization. Her style of dress is classic, and her personal flair comes through. Like any leader, she brings both professionalism and individuality to her job.

Perhaps the most difficult part of uniform dressing is to differentiate the female from the male version. They are equal but certainly not the same. The identifying factors have to do with style, color and fabric. It's not necessary for a woman to wear a female version of a man's suit to be in the corporate uniform. However, it is important to use the same cues: a suit with a matching skirt and jacket, a blouse in a solid color, and accessories that are simple and not distracting.

The team uniforms of the corporate world are not always the same. Their variety reflects the degree of tradition and conservatism of a particular team. However, the uniforms generally symbolize efficiency, organization and a sincere business attitude. These are desirable attributes in a Corporate profile.

At the most traditional end of the spectrum the uniform may

consist of very tailored, constructed clothing such as a matching navy or gray wool flannel suit with a blazer jacket and slim skirt. It is worn with a solid white or off-white blouse with a simple collar or a bow. Those women who enjoy wearing dresses may adapt the same conservative look with a simple, tailored shirtdress and jacket. As severe or somber as these outfits may sound, they can be made interesting by good style, good cut and good quality fabric. For example, the blazer jackets, slim skirts, and silk or cotton blouses made by designers such as Evan Picone or Stanley Blacker, while not inexpensive, nevertheless offer a classic cut, fabrication and tailoring that can last for years. The investment in these clothes can often be amortized over time, and the return, in terms of self-esteem and professional enhancement, may be well worth the money.

At the contemporary end of the spectrum, the Corporate uniform can be adapted with jackets that come in a variety of shapes from cardigan looks to double-breasted blazers. They may be made in wovens or knit fabrics, and the colors may range from black to navy, gray, wine, red, brown, beige or even white. The matching skirts may be slim, dirndl, pleated or A-lines. The blouses may be white, off-white or pale pastels, or even a bright color like yellow, red or royal blue. Dresses need not be only shirt styles but may include a number of different looks that are smart yet professional. Clothes designed by Ralph Lauren, Calvin Klein or Liz Claiborne generally fit in here.

Often women start out their careers by dressing in a traditional Corporate style and then change to a more contemporary look. This change may be immediate or gradual, depending upon how quickly you achieve credibility and how the other women in the organization dress.

Businesswomen are entitled to wear feminine clothing. An imitation of a man's suit generally looks like just that. After all, a woman's body is shaped differently from a man's, so why wear a suit made for a man's body? A woman's suit is cut to conform to a woman's body. That doesn't mean it should emphasize our curves or sexuality. It does mean, however, that it should be flattering. The jacket should have some shaping to it and may have some details of a man's jacket such as an inside pocket, handsewn buttonholes, or a well-constructed collar and lapels. The skirt should have enough flare and ease to allow you to walk comfortably, climb stairs easily and, if necessary, run for a taxi, bus or plane.

Let's meet several women whose jobs come under the Corporate profile. Each has a different style and works in a different field, yet all dress in an appropriate, feminine way that gives them a professional appearance.

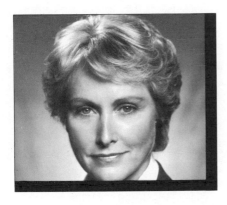

JUDY MAPES:
EXECUTIVE
RECRUITER

Judy Mapes provides an excellent example of the Corporate woman. She is a partner with Egon Zehnder International Inc., a management recruiting firm. She is currently the only woman on the company team, a team composed of eighty executive players. Her job is to help corporate clients identify and select candidates for top positions such as president or chief executive officer.

Mapes is a traditional dresser by nature and feels very comfortable dressing in the style that is also natural to her company. "This is a Swiss firm," she says. "It's a major international firm. It has a very high quality image, conducts very high management searches, but is very, very Swiss conservative. We don't hire anybody who doesn't have an MBA. It's basically a very elitist kind of firm and everybody here dresses accordingly. But," she explains, "that's because that's the way they normally dress. People who dress that way get hired by this firm. It's not that they change their dress when they get here."

She emphasizes her own conservative nature. "For me to dress trendy would be out of character . . . I wear mostly black, navy, gray. I buy good quality, reasonably priced, well-cut suits that fit. I buy about two suits a year . . . I like silk shirts in different colors. I have a hot pink one, but I'd only wear it if I didn't have a client meeting."

Although her office is in New York City, the center of the fashion industry, fashion is not a part of her image. In fact, she backs away from it. Mapes feels that if she dressed in high-fashion clothes, they would detract from the impression she wants to create of a serious Corporate executive. She believes that wearing such clothes implies she spends a lot of time and money on her appearance and gives too little attention to the business at hand.

Mapes says, "Quality clothes that fit, are pressed and well-cut are important. We charge very high fees, and I dress conservatively so that someone doesn't say, 'There goes my fee on her Chanel suit.'"

Indeed, her clothes have quite the opposite effect. That conservative side of her is what is most appealing to her firm and her clients. But don't for a moment think that Mapes is dowdy. She is a very attractive woman—tall and slim, and though her style is crisp, her look is decidedly Corporate chic.

Mapes almost always wears suits because they make her feel businesslike. She believes that when she wears dresses she is seen in a different light. "I feel much more social in a dress. I have a couple of very conservative silk dresses that I wear to work. But again, I don't wear them with clients. The dresses re-emphasize the fact I'm a female. A lot of what I do could be interpreted as social. I don't want anybody to think I'm there for social purposes. I'm not. I'm there for business. So I don't want to confuse anybody by what I say or how I look. If they have to pay a $50,000 fee, I want them to understand that every minute they spend with me is business."

The day we met she was wearing a simple, well-cut black gabardine suit from Saint Laurie, a New York manufacturer that makes suits for women as well as men. But Mapes' suit didn't look like a man's suit. It fit her well and showed off her lanky figure. The skirt had kick pleats which allowed her to cross her legs easily without being concerned about exposing her knees or thighs, a problem with some very narrow skirts. She could move well without feeling constrained. Although she usually wears silk blouses, that day she had on a simple white cotton pleated shirt. She wore it with the collar open. Around her neck was a gold necklace, and she wore black and gold earrings and a gold watch. Her hair was short and brushed away from her face. She wore a slight bit of makeup which was all that was necessary on her suntanned face.

Judy Mapes fits right in with the men in her organization who dress in conservative, dark business suits. Her look is precise, neat, professional and feminine. She spends very little time shopping. Her planned wardrobe strategy means she knows exactly what works. She uses one basic shopping resource where she refreshes her wardrobe for the season. She views her clothes as long-term investments: She is not interested in risky fads and wants a solid return.

KAREN VALENSTEIN: BANKER

When Karen Valenstein appeared on the cover of the *New York Times Magazine* she was dressed in a navy Chanel-style cardigan jacket. Inside the magazine, in a profile story about this first vice president of E. F. Hutton, she was photographed at lunch with three businessmen: the men all wore navy suits and she was wearing a single-breasted navy jacket. Karen Valenstein wears traditional clothes and varies them to fit her audience: tailored on some occasions, softer on others. She isn't afraid to add feminine details and uses pastel tweeds when replicating her original Chanel suits. The *Times,* calling her "one of the pre-eminent women in banking," says, "For Mrs. Valenstein, clothes are a tool of her trade that she wields like a master."

Although she strongly rejects rigid gray flannel and masculine bow ties, Valenstein wears structured suits when she's in cities like New York and San Francisco, and switches to casual clothes when she's in the country. She recognizes the suit as a symbol of professionalism yet makes sure hers have femininity and flair.

In the same article, other women in banking showed a similar attitude. Susan G. Fisher, senior vice president at Marine Midland Bank, was photographed wearing a black suit—the cardigan jacket was buttonless and trimmed with white. Myrna Weiss, marketing executive for Rothschild Inc., was shown wearing a black jacket over a red pleated dress. Both women looked competent and feminine: full-fledged, female members of their teams.

As Valenstein demonstrates, any single look is not always appropriate; the look may vary with your audience. One woman I interviewed talked about a friend of hers, Nancy, who is a lawyer. Nancy went shopping and bought four conservative suits when she began her career. But she has since found that her moods change and so do the attitudes of her clients. The friend explains, "There are days when Nancy does not want to be looked at, when she wants to be absorbed into the room of gray and blues, and there are other days when she wants to charm a little bit. On those days she'll wear a dress or a more feminine suit. She knows there are clients who want to hear that message. Nancy has a fashion client, a Seventh Avenue firm, and when they come in, she doesn't want to dress as if she doesn't know what they're talking about, so she styles it up a little bit."

SHELLEY BIGELMAN: ACCOUNT EXECUTIVE

Women who work for conservative companies must always make an extra effort to conform. Shelley Bigelman is a marketing manager at Lever Brothers. She oversees a category of products that includes dishwashing cleansers such as All and Sunlite, and has several account managers who report to her. Bigelman is one of the top women in the company and is very aware of her appearance. She says, "My company is very male. There are not many females here. I deal with upper management and staff groups—sales, manufacturing, research and development, promotion services and advertising agencies. One image you want to portray is just being a professional person. No one should notice the clothes you wear. Eighty percent of my work clothes are suits or skirts and jackets. For ease of wardrobe I use navy, gray, white and khaki."

Bigelman often wears bow ties with her blouses but has found that if she tries something more masculine it can backfire. A few times she wore a man's necktie. "My boss got very upset. He did not like those ties. I'd keep it slightly open with my collar open and a vest over it. He thought it was a very unfeminine way to dress." Bigelman's boss would define "professional" as appropriate and feminine. "You would never wear pants in my office," she says. "I wore pants to work once. The vice president of marketing said, 'I don't wear skirts to the office; you don't wear pants.'" Bigelman defines looking professional as saying to the onlooker, "Respect me." She doesn't want to appear distracting or have people think that other things interfere with business. "I don't want them to think that it took me two and one-half hours to get dressed. I want them to know that my number one priority is doing the best job."

It's important to be conscious of attitudes in your work community. What is acceptable in one office may not be acceptable in another, even in the same field. And what may be attractive to one person may be threatening to another. One woman told me about an incident in her law firm which surprised the women there but which taught them a useful lesson. One of the women in the firm wore a new bow tie to work one day and went in to talk to one of the senior partners. "She came out shaking her head. He was staring at her and staring at her and she couldn't figure out why. The next day he wore a tie made of the exact same silk." Now the women in that office tend to wear bow ties that are made of fabric other than that used for men's ties. Dressing like a man can be threatening to men. Dressing in tailored clothes with feminine touches is more readily acceptable.

Dressing in the Corporate mode, you also run the risk of looking too bland or boring. A recent article in the *New York Times* discussed how some students at Yale University dress for job interviews. The article said, "Job-hunting season has begun and every day investment banks and large corporations come to New Haven to interview seniors. Suddenly, clothing has become all-important. People usually seen in jeans are appearing at breakfast in suits and intently discussing the nuances of business attire, striving to project the proper image."

Many of the women were wearing dark suits, white blouses and conservative accessories. One woman said, "It's like playing the game." Another said, "It's kind of like you're buying a uniform." Another called her suit, which she hoped was seen as her commitment to the banking community, "the most boring piece of clothing ever."

These women are certainly aware of the need to adopt the team uniform. But they haven't learned how to let their individuality come through. It's true they shouldn't wear clothing which detracts from what they have to say. But they are equally mistaken to assume that companies want to hire bland, neutered people. You don't want to be outrageous in the way you dress; however you won't lose points for making an attractive, distinctive appearance either.

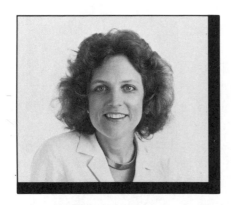

BETH MILWID:
CORPORATE
PSYCHOLOGIST

There are other types of jobs within the corporate world that have even more leeway. Beth Milwid is at the contemporary end of the Corporate range. She is a psychologist who has been featured on the cover of *Savvy* magazine for her research on the feelings of women who work in male-dominated industries. She was hired as a consultant to the Crocker Bank in San Francisco and decided to play by the team rules.

Milwid says, "When I came to the bank it was very important that I wear a navy blue suit. A lot of the women there were wearing navy blue suits and black pinstripe suits. We used to laugh and call ourselves 'bankerettes'."

Although she may have laughed at her uniform, it helped identify her as a member of the team. Since her position as a psychologist was not a traditional line job in banking, she had an uphill battle to fight. Many of the bank people were suspicious of her, and she had to establish her credibility quickly. Dressing the way they did, communicating in their clothing language, was important.

Milwid found, however, that the uniform need not be so restrictive. "You don't have to wear blue," she says now. "You can wear blue, and you can mix it with some soft touches. I'm not saying everyone should wear pink . . . I'm saying find out who you are and be it. And don't threaten anybody. Join them. Tell them what you can offer, and tell them you <u>want</u> to learn what they've got to offer."

Although Milwid believes there is a shift away from the strict navy suit and towards more individual dressing, she thinks it will be a while before major changes take place in an industry as conservative as banking. Bankers are not ready for Victorian style dresses, clinging knits and women in pants. "You don't have to have black, you don't have to have navy. But err in that direction for a while. Play your game but do it in a subtle way. They're not ready for screamers. The framework is go slow to go fast."

She gives this advice to women who resist dressing in the Corporate profile. "Someone once told me there are only two things you really have to realize to be successful in a corporation. At the first cut, show up every day for work on time, and dress to play the game. I'm saying that's only the beginning, but if you don't dress to play the game—this is a visual culture—they look at you and they say, 'go or no go'. And you're 'no go'. No matter what, you can't get in. This is critical for women. You have to understand the rules of your industry and your company. Look around, press the edges as to your new contribution as a woman, but understand that in banking you dress differently than in Hollywood. Dress—it's very, very, very important. It's *the* issue in corporations."

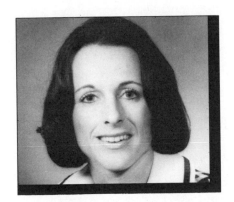

CINDY RYAN:
ATTORNEY

Cindy Ryan is a successful California attorney who has moved from one end of the spectrum of Corporate dressing to the other. When I first met her several years ago, she was very traditional in her appearance. Her hair was short, she wore glasses, used very little makeup, and dressed mostly in navy suits. Recently we met again, and when I saw the woman at the door, I wasn't sure it was Cindy Ryan. True, it was a Sunday afternoon in the summer, but she looked like an entirely different person. Her hair was long and full, she did not have on glasses, she wore makeup and hot pink lipstick, and was dressed in a bright turquoise, crinkly cotton jumpsuit.

When Ryan graduated from law school and interviewed for jobs, she dressed in a traditional style. She kept that look for the first few years of her career and believes that it helped establish her credibility as a serious lawyer. She stayed away from anything blatantly feminine, yet she wore clothes that were well-cut and made for a woman.

She says, "I wore black Evan Picone suits with white blouses, very little jewelry, and looked pretty nondescript. The message I was trying to get across was, 'You are not hiring anything but a capable lawyer.' I was trying to get across that you would not be influenced by anything I was wearing, that I had a neutral look." Of course, whatever we wear has an influence. What she achieved was a look of professionalism and appropriateness without letting her clothes be distracting.

She believes that it is always important to wear the proper costume for the role you are playing. She has become aware of how clothing affects people's perception of her. She learned the hard way that the obvious may not always be the most effective way to look. "Essentially what we're talking about is dressing for the occasion and what works. I learned in a couple of instances what didn't work. I often had evening events to go to, and early on I would attend them on behalf of the company, and my husband would accompany me. In those circumstances, sometimes I would wear a cocktail dress which was appropriate for the event. But unfortunately, many, many times, before I was known in those circles, people would come up—especially political candidates—and say to my husband, 'Thank you, Mr. Ryan, for helping us this evening', when I was, in fact, the person to thank. That happened because my dress was more that of a wife than a business person. So, in many instances, when it said 'cocktail' I would dress in a business suit just like all the other men who had raced from their job and didn't have time to change or freshen up. I learned my lesson."

Over the past few years, Ryan has made her style more contemporary. Now she adds more color and feminine touches and has learned to adapt her outfits to her audience. "I've also noticed that when I deal with rough and tumble entrepreneurs, especially in the real estate field, I tend to dress a little bit differently. I find that they are a little uncomfortable if you look too polished, too pinstripe-oriented. So I tend to dress a little bit more with color, not necessarily flamboyant, but something that makes them feel a little more comfortable. It may be dressing in a slightly different way, let's say a khaki suit instead of navy blue or black or gray." One favorite outfit is a gray full skirted suit which she wears with a bright red blouse. She'll even top it with a big brimmed hat, an accessory she has come to enjoy.

Ryan views her traditional type of Corporate dressing as typical of women lawyers across the country. "The court system requires it," she says. "Not just the corporation and that setting, but the law firms do too. Although California is viewed as a fairly casual state, the major law firms still want you to dress in accordance with decor. When you go into federal court you'd have to be unobservant not to recognize that it's a very formal setting. If you're not dressed appropriately, it's going to affect the decision-making process."

Nevertheless, Ryan no longer believes that her appearance must be boring. She has changed jobs and now works for a private law firm. She wears suits that have more flair, blouses that have more color and adds amusing accessories when the mood moves her. She says, "Over the last few years I have gained credibility. People know what I do. I'm a partner in a major law firm that has been around for 60 years in California, which is old by California standards. About two or three years ago, I decided that I really didn't need, for the most part, to always dress in the uniform. I felt like I was being regimented. The uniform was a symbol of my credibility and competence, my acceptance into the legal profession; it said that I was equal to anybody in the field. Now my credits speak for themselves. So the fact that I dress to please myself now, in many instances, becomes irrelevant. I feel better about it, because it really reflects my personality. On the other hand, when I go into government, and I do a lot of work with the government, I tend to dress down again. The difference is that now, instead of wearing a white blouse, I tend to wear a lot of pinks, a lot of turquoise, and other more flamboyant colors."

To emphasize her femininity, she has even refurnished her office. When she began her law career, her office was in keeping with the masculine looks around her. Now she uses softer, more feminine fabrics. Ryan's change took time. She waited until she felt confident that her reputation was established. Now she enjoys letting her personality show through in her style but still stays within the Corporate profile.

THE SUBTLE DIFFERENCES. The styles of career dressing change not just from job to job, but within the same job. In the field of law, for example, attorneys who have reached a level of success where they are appearing before the Supreme Court have been known to call the Court to find out how to dress. A source inside the Supreme Court is quoted in an article in the *Legal Times* of Washington, D.C., as saying that, "Many lawyers call the Clerk's office prior to oral argument for guidance on proper attire. The Clerk may also check lawyers for correct dress before they enter the courtroom. Dark suits with white shirts and subdued ties or scarves are considered most appropriate." This same source observes that "Most lawyers who come before the Court follow the rules," but adds that there is a small group of lawyers who appear frequently before the Court and they "go the extra mile to appear immaculately tailored and they do stand out from the crowd." The article concludes, "Superior appearance communicates both confidence in one's argument and courtesy towards the Court."

There is no doubt that your appearance communicates how you feel about yourself and your audience. But courtroom lawyers are not always addressing the Justices of the Supreme Court. Sometimes they are appearing in front of a judge and sometimes in front of a judge and jury. In each case, your appearance may differ.

In a survey taken by researchers from Brigham Young University and Virginia Polytechnic Institute and reprinted in *Harper's Magazine,* the question was asked, "In an area as steeped in ceremony as the courtroom, just what should the female lawyer wear in order to appear convincing? Because judges, colleagues, and jurors are as easily influenced by appearances as the rest of the populace, clothing credibility is a crucial support to a good argument or the conduct of any aspect of a case." The researchers surveyed 100 former jurors and stated: "Our research has found that a woman lawyer may confidently select a tailored suit and blouse as appropriate for courtroom wear, but attention to such accessories as neckwear is warranted." Their findings showed that a soft bow or soft scarf tucked inside the jacket were the most effective looks for conveying authority. The least effective was the controversial menswear bow tie. Said the researchers, "That might be explained by the possible masculine impression created by this tie's crispness."

Authority, however, may not be the only attribute you want to suggest to a jury. Some lawyers use clothing cues that identify them with the jury. Attorneys have been known to wear boots because the foreman wore boots, or to wear a certain color because that was a color worn by several members of the jury. Defense attorneys may sometimes want to look slightly more casual, inferring a link with the jury rather than with the prosecution. On the other hand, prosecuting attorneys may want to appear more authoritative and serious. Small details, such as the color of your blouse or the style of your earrings, can have an amazing impact on your appearance. In all cases, this silent communication through clothing can have an important effect on the courtroom audience.

Whether in a courtroom or a corporation, the psychological impact of appearance is undeniable. The more familiar you are with what your clothes communicate, the more you can use them to your advantage. The more comfortable you are with your appearance, the more you communicate confidence and competence.

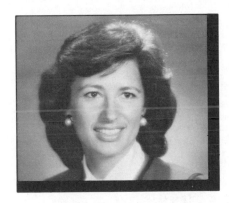

JULIETTE HEINTZE: FINANCIER

Juliette Heintze is an executive who telegraphs confidence and an attractive appearance. She has changed her style of dress as she has moved within the field of finance from banking to corporate life. She is the treasurer of USAir, the only female officer of this billion dollar plus airline. She started out her career in banking in New York City, first with Chase Manhattan and then with Manufacturers Hanover Trust. Now she is based in Virginia. Looking back she says, "At that time there were very few women in corporate lending so there were no role models. I was surrounded by men in navy blue or dark gray three piece suits. I think when you represent a conservative institution you do tend to dress differently than when you're working for a corporation like I am now. I tend to think of a woman representing a bank having a need to be more conservative—maybe her colors a little more subdued and the cut of her clothes more classic—than women in advertising or marketing." She favors clothes from Albert Nipon, Liz Claiborne and St. Tropez but says, "I do not buy clothes by label. What attracts me first is fabric, then color and style."

She wears suits and dresses and always makes sure that the dresses are accompanied by a jacket. "I do think jackets are an important part of a wardrobe. Somehow, wearing a jacket equates to being one of the guys. I've noticed lately at staff meetings we'll all go in with our suits on, and then the guys will take off their jackets, or I'll take off my jacket. Somehow, a jacket is a great equalizer in a wardrobe."

Although within the company there is little emphasis on clothing, this financial manager believes it can be a big asset when used effectively. "I really don't think clothes play a big role at USAir. I really don't think senior management cares what I wear as long as I look neat and respectable," Heintze says. "But I do think it's a valuable tool. It sets the tone."

She sees a definite advantage in the variety of women's clothing and uses different looks at different times. "Women have a lot more flexibility in this than men do, so I think it's an advantage. If I know I'm going to be leading a meeting, I'll tend to wear a navy suit and a white shirt. I think about the jewelry I'm wearing. I might wear small pierced earrings."

She favors colors such as grays, browns and beiges, and chooses them in solids or tweeds. "I occasionally throw in some nice bright blouses to break up the darker suits," she says. "Sometimes I like to wear a red silk blouse with a gray flannel suit." But Heintze doesn't always wear a suit. The day we met she was wearing a royal blue silk dress with a jacket. "Now that I'm in a corporation I feel I have a little more freedom in my wardrobe. Now I'm a customer. They are calling on *me*. The banks are coming here, calling on the company. Now my responsibility is not to represent a conservative bank but to represent a successful corporation."

Whether she wears a suit or a dress and jacket, Heintze makes sure she feels comfortable in her clothes and is appropriately attired. She says, "I learned something once and it was very important to me. It was to always wear something that you would be happy wearing to lunch if somebody called you up spontaneously and just said, 'Let's have lunch today'. That really worked wonders for me. I think that's one of my basic creeds now." Like many women she admits, "I used to sneak things just for the sake of wearing them. Sure enough, that would be the day somebody would call me. I said, 'I'm not going to do this anymore'. If you look good, you feel good about yourself."

Knowing the right looks to include in your Corporate wardrobe will make dressing a great deal easier for you. Your wardrobe can help you feel good about the way you look, and give you the confidence to communicate your competence and femininity. In Chapter VI we show you several different ways to put together a Corporate Capsule.

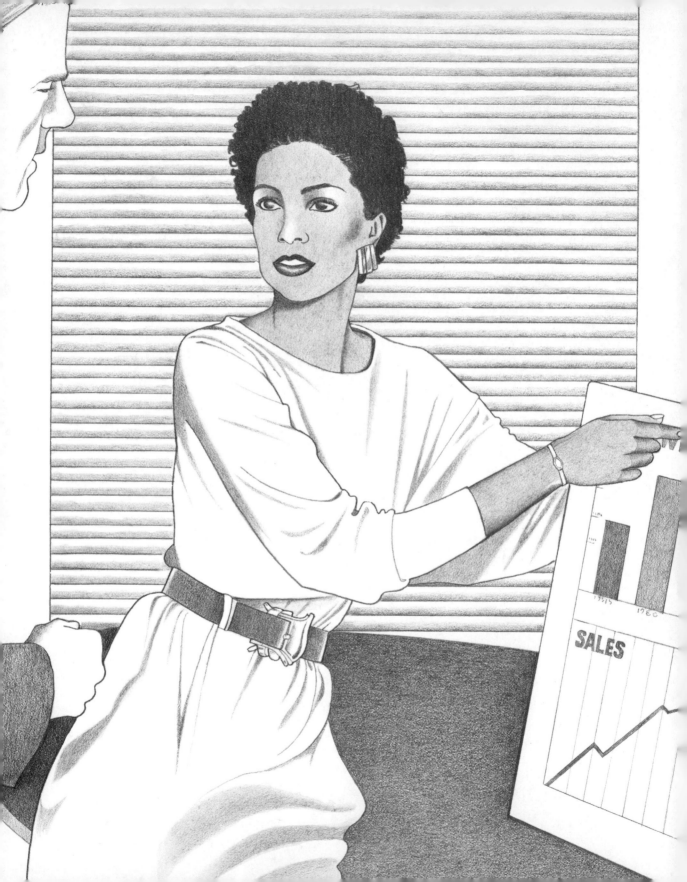

CHAPTER III

The Communicator Profile

Men have traditionally succeeded by climbing the corporate ladder. Women, however, are discovering other routes. Indeed, it may very well be because of the predominance of men in the traditional corporate world that women are searching to establish themselves in other fields. While the doors of the corporate com-

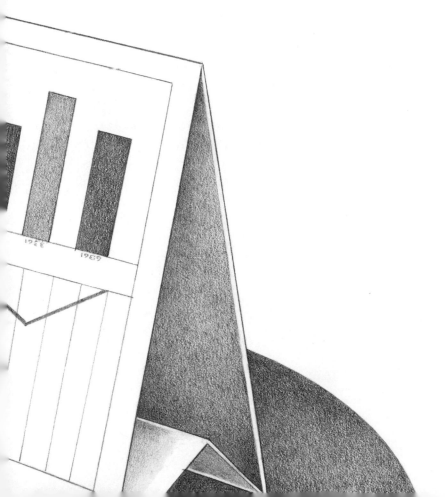

munity have been closed to many women, other areas are more welcoming, offer more entry level placements and more opportunities for advancement. Some fields, such as education and retailing, have been filled with women for many years. But now women are making deeper inroads and exploring new paths in previously untouched territories. These paths may lead to careers in fields as varied as advertising, sales and marketing, media, small business ownership, fund-raising, politics, public relations, or clinical psychology and sociology.

As diverse and disparate as these careers may seem, there are several factors that unite them under the umbrella of the Communicator profile. They all stress sincerity, friendliness, persuasiveness, and a relationship with people who are outside the immediate organization. These relationships are essential to career development. If you are already in any of these fields or are considering entering one of them, you probably are aware that a person-to-person relationship is the basis for growth in your career. Your success is determined by outward reach. Whether as a sales representative for a computer company, an account executive for an advertising agency, or a teacher in a classroom, the key to success is building and maintaining a relationship with your audience. As a sales representative, your audience is your customer. As an account executive, your audience is your client. And as a teacher, your student. In each of these areas, your audience is outside your organization, and you must extend yourself out to it to achieve what you want.

The key phrases in a Communicator profile are personal relationships and outward reach. Implicit in these ideas are the elements of accessibility, sincerity and an interest in the other person's needs. The very word "communicate" suggests a give and take, an exchange of information and ideas. Unlike the upwardly mobile corporate world, which focuses on facts rather than friendships, efficiency over emotion, the world of the Communicator is based on convincing an outside audience of your sincerity and care in their concerns. To be a successful teacher, you must be understanding of your students, yet firm in imparting information. To be a successful sales executive, you must show understanding of your client's needs, yet be assertive in establishing your product's value. That's how you gain an audience's appreciation and respect.

The Communicator profile also contains important elements of persuasion and knowledge. To achieve real success and establish a continuing relationship with your customers and clients, they must believe that first, you understand their needs and have their best interests at heart; second, you know your product well; and third, because of these factors, you know if your product is right for them. It doesn't matter what your product is; it may be new math, negligees or the nightly news. Irrespective, you must present it thoroughly and convincingly, at the same time showing knowledge of your audience's need for your product.

The Communicator profile covers a wide variety of fields and occupations. Many of the jobs are in sales and service areas that are comfortable for many women.

Counsels Beth Milwid, "We're moving towards a more sectored economy and an information-based economy. Women have shmoozed on the phone with their girlfriends for a hundred years . . . so women have strengths based on socializing." In other words, use your abilities to make friends, talk to people and spread the news, and turn those skills into assets to help advance your career.

Skills that come naturally to women are often more difficult for men. As a result, David King, founder of Careers for Women, concludes, "More women will enter the executive boardroom through the 'sales' door than from graduate programs in law and business combined." He emphasizes that it is in the areas of executive sales, where personal relationships are built and business is on a repeat basis, that women stand out. These areas include real estate, which traditionally has attracted women, advertising, insurance, securities and financing. King sees executive selling as an ideal area for women since it is an occupation where socializing is essential for building continuing relationships with clients. "You don't just talk about your product and your service, you talk about your client's vacation, your client's dog, your dog. It's social conversation. At those levels of friend-making, women are so much better at it. Men tend to be monosyllabic. The average woman, when she meets a stranger, gets the stranger talking about himself. The average man tells the stranger about himself."

Women are finding success not just in selling but in the whole entrepreneurial area. They are establishing their own businesses and enjoying enormous rewards. According to the Small Business Administration, there are three million businesses owned by women, a number which has increased 69 percent in the ten years between 1972 and

1982. Charlotte Taylor, who writes a business column in *Working Woman* magazine, believes that this trend towards small business ownership by women is nothing less than a revolution in the American economy.

That same socializing aptitude, so effective in selling, also works well when you are trying to start a new company. If you are going to be successful in building a business, you must be able to persuade your audience of your ability, your knowledge and your interest in them. Managerial and organizational strengths, sometimes taken for granted in the home, are valuable tools in the business world.

SELLING YOURSELF

Selling yourself is the key to all of the occupations in the Communicator profile. That is perhaps best illustrated in the world of television, where audience ratings determine success or failure. On camera you must establish a rapport with your audience while demonstrating your knowledge of the subject matter. That means reaching out to win their confidence and support. After all, the audience must like and respect you if you are to gain their backing, and they must be able to identify with you in some meaningful way. Otherwise they will literally switch you off. There is no doubt that the television audience, like most audiences anywhere, would prefer watching someone who has an attractive, cheery appearance than someone who does not. That applies to male personalities as well as to female, and to guest appearances of all kinds.

Likewise in the area of education, whether the position involves teaching kindergarten children or college-age adults, the combination of friendliness and assertiveness is important for success. Whether students are five, fifteen or twenty-five, they respond positively to an open and attractive appearance. Young children often comment aloud on a teacher's colorful outfit or new dress; older students may simply emulate the style. Students of all ages look up to their teachers as role models. Every teacher has a ready audience. It is up to her to communicate with that audience.

When a sales agent meets a customer, a television personality appears on camera, or a teacher stands before a class, instant judgments are made about them, particularly about the way they look. In the opening seconds, when you are either accepted or rejected, appearance is everything. That may be unfair and somewhat shortsighted, but it is reality. Even if you have special talents and abilities, you have to work extra hard at your job if you lose your audience at the initial contact.

As a Communicator, you must dress to your audience and your message. There are certain clothing cues to be aware of. For example, your appearance should indicate an accessability, not intimidation, and it should express authority without being authoritarian. The severe, somber, structured business suit may be too stand-offish. The Communicator may still wear a suit, but it should be one that has more color, fabric interest or relaxed styling. The jacket, which is the symbol of authority to the Corporate woman, may not be used in the same way by a Communicator. When it is used, it doesn't always match the skirt or dress, and may be constructed or unconstructed. The matched suit, a power image in the corporate world, may be the wrong packaging for the Communicator. Instead of acting as a connector, it cuts you off from your audience. Colors and patterns the Communicator chooses may be broader in range and brighter in tone. Fabrics may be more varied, emphasize softer wovens or fluid knits. There is also greater choice in styles which range from updated to more innovative. Much of this depends upon you, your product and your audience.

COMMUNICATING ON CAMERA

Television may be at once the most difficult and the most powerful medium to conquer. To be effective on television requires an enormous amount of poise and confidence combined with a solid understanding of the subject and an appearance that is attractive without being distracting.

Diane Sawyer, the only woman journalist on the news program "60 Minutes," has said that it is very important that a woman look "complete." That complete look usually comes with wearing a jacket or a tailored dress, and suggests authority and assertiveness. She emphasizes the importance of not being distracting on camera. The danger lies in losing the audience as they focus on your jewelry, your hair or your dress instead of paying attention to your words.

In studies conducted at Texas Tech University, audiences were asked to watch television news anchorwomen who were dressed in three different styles: conservative, trendy and casual. The conservative look, which meant a navy jacket and striped bow neck blouse, was the most effective. They found that there was a significant difference in the retention of material by audiences depending upon the way the newscaster was dressed. The less finished and more informal the outfit, the more the audience was distracted.

At the same time that authority is expressed in the newscaster's outfit, her appearance should suggest some softness and femininity. A harsh or strident look will also "turn off" many viewers. The newscaster must communicate the serious events in the news to an audience relaxing at home. In effect, she straddles two different worlds.

The women in this chapter represent a variety of Communicator profiles. Each person pays attention to her audience's needs and combines this with individual flair.

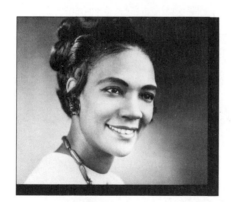

FREDDIE LUCAS: GOVERNMENT RELATIONS REPRESENTATIVE

When you hear the word "sales," you may think of a woman behind a counter or an Avon representative. But selling can denote a world of different products and audiences. It can mean selling cosmetics to the customer at home, or it can mean selling the interests of an industry to Congressional legislators. This second area, commonly known as lobbying, is an influential occupation in the nation's capital. Many large companies have their own staff lobbyists, while numerous other organizations around the country hire local

Washington public relations firms to lobby for them. The women in these positions, who are actively working at persuading an audience of traditionalists in government, must dress in a way that is attractive and feminine, but never flamboyant.

Freddie Hill Lucas is a senior representative for industry-government relations for the General Motors Corporation. Her job is to persuade legislators to act in the interests of her company. Lucas, who is an attractive black woman, married, and the mother of three children, is also on the boards of the YWCA, the Industrial Research Relations Association, and the American League of Lobbyists.

Her working wardrobe often functions for very long days, beginning with breakfast on Capitol Hill and moving on to meetings, lunches, more meetings, cocktail receptions and dinner parties. When Lucas dresses in the morning, she must be aware of her company, her audience and her own personal style. She compares herself with G.M. "General Motors is successful and my appearance can be no less so. It's a quiet, conservative company that will always recognize its tremendous opportunities in its future. It's a very vital company so I want to show vitality. It's a very solid company so I want to give an appearance of strength in my fashion and my look. I want the General Motors image and me to be compatible." Lucas says she enjoys her clothes, likes to look attractive, but adds, "I don't want to bowl you over."

The day Lucas and I met, she was dressed in a lilac Ultra-suede suit and a cream colored blouse. With it she wore an ivory necklace which set off the outfit beautifully. Typically, she wears suits or dresses and jackets in a broad range of colors that includes black, gray, navy, brown, beige, maroon and lilac. Since her suits are fairly simple in style, she's always looking for new and interesting blouses to wear with them. "It's very important to have lots of different blouses," she says. Lucas also mixes her skirts and jackets, rather than staying with only matched suits, and enhances her clothes with African jewelry. Because she goes from high-powered meetings to social affairs, she relies on dark colors which look elegant in the evening as well as during the day. She describes her black suits as high-powered and high-fashion "without knocking anyone down."

Knocking someone down is about the last thing she wants to do. If Lucas' image were too strong, too strident or flamboyant, she would offend her traditional audience. But she does want them to remember her and think of her as representative of her company. She must project the successful image of the nation's largest auto maker. Her appearance must be professional, but with the femininity and softness that allows her audience to identify with her and relate to her as a friend. Lucas' suits and blouses or dresses and jackets give her authority and femininity, and her jewelry both reflects her personality and also offers a conversational opening, the perfect combination for a Communicator.

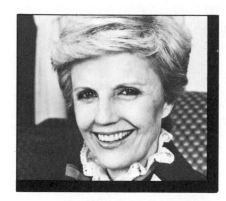

N A N C Y R E Y N O L D S : L O B B Y I S T

W hile Freddie Hill Lucas is on the staff of a large corporation, other lobbyists, such as Nancy Reynolds and Anne Wexler, have their own public relations firms which represent a number of different clients. Both women, who are political opposites but partners together in their own company, give a good deal of thought to their image. Like most successful women, they have little time to devote to shopping. They like high-quality clothing and are sensitive to their various audiences' levels of dress.

Reynolds says, "We represent clients who are relatively conservative and expect businesslike and professional behavior out of us. So we wear what we think are well-cut, nice looking clothes, but nothing they would ever remark on. I wear very, very conservative things on the Hill."

Her days are not always spent with Congressmen and Senators. She may be meeting with long-time clients, making presentations to new clients, delivering speeches, or attending any of the constant breakfasts, lunches and dinners that consume Washington life. Her look may change, depending upon her agenda. She may dress quietly in conservative navy or go all out with a high-fashion raspberry Chanel suit and matching blouse.

As for the raspberry suit she says, "I'd wear it to a cocktail party, I'd wear it to give a speech, I'd wear it to make a presentation." However, she avoids expensive fashion symbols when she is on the Hill. "I would never lobby in a fur coat. I think it says you're showing off a lot of money. You're dealing with people who certainly never make more than $30,000 or $40,000 a year. I think you have to remember whom you're going to talk to."

Reynolds had previously worked for the Bendix Corporation and has always been cautious about her appearance in the corporate world. Although she dressed in some bright colors she never looked flamboyant, which she would consider inappropriate. "I don't think reeking of chic is very businesslike here or in the corporate world," she says, speaking of Washington ways. "When you are dealing with people during the day, you're sending a message . . . I think you have to be careful when you're lobbying. You're dealing with a lot of people. You want them to remember what you've said, not what you look like."

Reynolds and Wexler do not confuse careful with dull. Their styles are neither bland nor drab. As entrepreneurial women, eager to build their business and make their mark, they both want to be recognizable. They feel there is plenty of room for their own personalities to come through. Says Reynolds, "I think as I grew older and became more confident, I felt less bound. I wear lots of bright colors. They not only make me feel terrific, but I look well in clear bright red, clear blue, clear yellow. So I wear them to please myself now."

Both women are aware of the effect of their dressing on potential clients. They know that wearing good quality, well-cut, well-styled clothes suggests that they are successful. Their implicit message is that those who hire them will be successful too.

Reynolds often wears knit suits and usually adds a jacket to separate skirts. "Jackets are very important," she says. The day we talked she was wearing a wine-colored cardigan sweater over a navy skirt and white blouse. "I probably wouldn't be wearing this sweater today if I were having a client meeting," she explains, "because I think a jacket is more serious." She compares the way she dresses for different occasions, noting that there are times when the Communicator can adapt the uniform of the Corporate woman without looking too severe. "If I were giving a formal presentation to new clients, I would probably wear a suit, unless it was a tailored dress that I liked very much, or a knit suit. I'm very fond of knit suits. We certainly consider them on the same level as a regular (woven) suit. They're very feminine too. I think that's the great thing about them. You're in the prescribed uniform but knit suits are soft and comfortable and obviously feminine without being noticeably or markedly feminine."

AMANDA HAHN: ACCOUNT EXECUTIVE

While Lucas, Reynolds and Wexler are smoothing the way for their clients on Capitol Hill, Amanda Hahn is selling the consumer from her office on Madison Avenue. She is now a senior account executive with N. W. Ayer and had been with Benton and Bowles, whose clients include major consumer product manufacturers such as Colgate Palmolive. Prior to joining an advertising agency she interviewed with several large companies, including both manufacturers and ad agencies. Hahn says that her decision was partly affected by the way people dressed in the different organizations. She compares the two sides of the consumer products industry: "The client side tends to be fairly conservative. It still has dark suits with ties at the throat, whereas advertising is a whole lot freer."

Advertising agencies act as great communicators, selling to both their clients and the consumer while straddling the worlds of the corporate and the creative. Hahn describes Benton and Bowles as a traditional company; however, its role as a "Communicator" company prescribes that dressing not be so conservative. "Benton and Bowles is a very marketing, old boy, eastern establishment kind of place. You'll find a range here, but certainly more freedom than you get with our clients.

You can see a broad range of people walking through the halls, but really a minimum of standard MBA uniform."

Because their corporate audience has its dress code, account executives adapt that look for client meetings and presentations. As Communicators, they are eager to speak the same language as their audience. Says Hahn, "The suit says, 'It's what I know they'll be wearing.' I think it's the same way you match what the client's doing in a whole lot of hierarchical ways, business ways . . . I can get away with looking different internally, and get the proper response out of people. But I think the client expects you a certain way. It's really a double standard. I think internally you can turn people off by looking too businesslike, because advertising is an industry where you have to be more creative, a little freer, looser. I want to convey that kind of impression to people."

Hahn prefers sportswear and dresses to matched suits and laughs at the memory of being trained at business school to dress in the Corporate uniform. She says, "I really have no great love of a suit. I don't own any of those little ties for the throat." Even the suits she does own are soft, unconstructed, and have interesting patterns and textures.

She sees her own style of dress as typical of the company. "There are a few people who are very tailored, the standard business look, but that's not really the way around here. That was brought home to me when I was waiting to go into a meeting and a woman walked out in the whole blue suit look. Someone said, 'Who is that?' She was new, I explained. They said, 'No wonder she looks like that.' That's really the feeling. They expect a little more interesting dress. . . . It's that fine line, nothing that's ever non-professional, but we don't look like bankers."

Before going with Benton and Bowles, Hahn was with another New York advertising agency which was a "medium to large, medium-sized firm and is now a small–large firm." The company's image has changed along with its client list. When she worked there several years ago, she says, "Leather pants were appropriate for people who worked in my job as an account executive. . . . now they hire people who wear silk ties because they have a very different kind of client and they think that's what their client wants."

She explains how the clients have changed. "R. J. Reynolds was their major client. I think they liked the idea they were getting something a little stylish. I was working on More Lights, which is a woman's cigarette. I think they felt more comfortable feeling they had people with a little style. They're now working with Campbell's soup and more conservative clients. I think they're trying to pull in a more conservative market image."

In the advertising business as in all areas of selling, the successful account executive or salesperson speaks the language of her clients. Were the account executive to dress at odds with her client, there would be little credibility to her sales pitch. She would be alienating herself. By reflecting the client's look, she immediately establishes a bond.

At the same time, as a Communicator she has the freedom to express her personality and the agency's image—which generally stresses a creative approach.

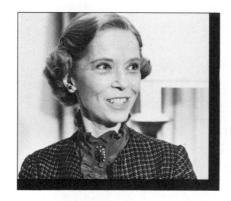

JEAN SISCO: ENTREPRENEUR

Women who have their own businesses, whether as a one woman consultant or as owner of a company, are entrepreneurs who come under the Communicator profile. Jean Sisco is a corporate consultant who has reached the rare heights of being on the boards of major corporations such as Carter Hawley Hale Stores, which owns the Broadway department stores in California, Neiman-Marcus, and Bergdorf Goodman; Textron; United Brands and many others. She has her own company and spends a good portion of her time traveling around the country.

Sisco has a strong background in retailing, having spent twenty-five years working for Marshall Field's and later Woodward & Lothrop. Her style of dress expresses her fashion background. While she would not be called flamboyant, she does show flair and individuality. She considers her appearance to be part and parcel of her overall product.

"I think dressing right is another skill," she says. "Correct speech, delivery, writing skills, reading skills, all of these are important. Think of all the money we spend on advertising products, on design, on color, on packaging." Sisco believes it is essential to have a "put-together appearance that relates well to our product and sells our product, whether it's a material product or a service, it's all part of the whole ambience of doing business."

Sisco's personal packaging includes her signature hats, classic clothes and low-keyed jewelry. She enjoys wearing colors and wants to be seen as attractive and feminine. "Since the men are dressed in the grays, the blues, the blacks and the browns, I tend to wear something that has color in it. I think I am different. I am a woman. I think that emphasizing the positive, and flattering it, is the way to go rather than trying to hide it. You're not going to disguise that fact, and by attempting to disguise it, I think men will feel that either you have no self-confidence, or you aren't satisfied with your own image. Consequently, I think you've blown the whole thing."

She received her first advice on professional dressing when she began working as a buyer at Marshall Field's in Chicago. "I remember one of the store's top buyers saying, 'Never wear anything that jingles', which was very good advice, because it's distracting. 'And nothing that wiggles, yourself or your clothes'. This to me is still good advice. I think that there is a certain sense of decorum that's necessary. But I think there is enough that is fashionable and well-chosen, even if you're worried about the properness of your outfit. I still think that people notice this; I notice it all the time when people come in to make their pitch. I figure if their self-esteem is high, they look good."

Being attractively dressed doesn't necessarily mean having pretty features or a gorgeous face. We can't all look like Raquel Welch but we can make the best of what we do have. Says Sisco, "Some of the ugliest women I've ever met have been some of the best dressed and the smartest. The smart woman is the woman who just steps a little bit ahead and has a little bit of a keynote or a signature of her own. That makes a difference. And you notice it. You really notice it."

Because she has her own consulting business, she is constantly selling herself. And she wants to make sure that she is perceived as a successful product. She packages herself in the most flattering colors and accents her outfits with fine jewelry. With her red hair and fair complexion, she favors colors like golds and greens. If she wears a navy suit, as she did on the day we talked, she'll brighten it with a turquoise blouse and antique turquoise and gold jewelry.

Sisco's audience is mostly male and highly successful. They are corporate presidents and chief executive officers who are very image conscious. She believes they appreciate good clothing for themselves and their peers. "I think men basically want their associates to look well. They expect it of one another. But we have so much wider a choice. Women have a lot of things. I think it's just another facet. If I didn't have any brains, and didn't know what I was doing, they could care less about how I looked. But I think they do like that additional side to my being a woman."

SUSAN MEYER: PUBLICIST

Susan Meyer is a Communicator who speaks to beauty and fashion editors at newspapers and magazines. She is an account executive with Ogilvy & Mather, a large public relations firm in New York, and represents clients like Louis Vuitton who are in fashion related areas. Meyer is extremely self-confident about her appearance and says, "I know what my style is. I am so confident that no matter the occasion I can easily determine what is the design or the style for me." Meyer is keenly aware of the message she wants her audience to receive. "I want them to think that I am fairly intelligent. I guess the word that I like is elegant. I'm not coy. That's not me. If I walk into a room I'd like to be thought of as an elegant person."

She has been aware of her own style for years, but what she

likes is to look "unstudied." Meyer says, "I don't want to look as though I have a hanger under my jacket and a label on the outside. This is my suit and it's my look and it's very important to me."

The clothes Meyer wears are mostly knits and often suits. Her favorite designer is Adolfo. She has worn his designs for many years and always feels comfortable in them. She believes a woman on a limited budget must first decide on her own look and then decide on "the colors that are best on you. Let's face it," she says, "you're not going to be able to afford thirty-two skirts. I would advise any woman on a limited budget to concentrate on separates, not dresses. A dress is a one-shot. You cannot wear it every day. But you can have two skirts and alternate them every other day and have totally different looks by changing off different sweaters and blouses, scarves and other accessories." She advises mixing the clothes from various manufacturers such as Liz Claiborne, Jones New York and Anne Klein. "Frivolity is something you can't afford," she says, "unless it's with an inexpensive accessory."

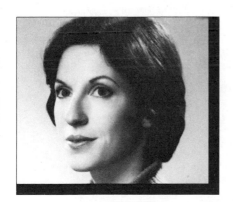

SUZANNE GARMENT:
JOURNALIST

Journalists are not generally admired for the way they dress; in fact, just the opposite. But television has changed that to some extent, and now you can see attractively dressed women reporters vying for the President's attention at nationally televised news conferences and on television talk shows.

Although the newspaper or magazine reporter doesn't often have to face a large group of people, you do have an audience, and that audience is the person you are interviewing. As a reporter, your credibility is helped or hindered by your appearance. Your ability to elicit information and to encourage confidence may depend to a great extent on the way you look. If a reporter dresses in a way that is at odds with the interviewee, there may be a real communication gap. The successful reporter establishes a rapport between herself and her interviewee, and part of that link comes by dressing in the same language.

Suzanne Garment is associate editor for the editorial page and columnist for the *Wall Street Journal*. She notices a difference in the way people in her office look depending upon their agenda for the day. Often they look casual, not far removed from their old college campus. But from time to time they will come to work looking more polished, more mature. She says, "When they have something important to do, like an interview, they feel they have to dress up. . . . I think when they dress up, it's wanting to be treated respectfully by the important people they are going to be with."

Garment calls casual clothing, such as skirts and sweaters or pants and shirts, "kidwear" because it reflects a younger, somewhat immature attitude. She dresses in a more grown-up style but is careful not to be too dressed up. She describes her own look as "somewhere between a working journalist and a lady type." Her appearance, naturally, is affected by her lifestyle which must take into account more than her career; it includes her husband, a prominent attorney, and their young daughter. "I'm married to someone who's older, and there's a whole part of my life that's running an establishment. On the other hand, I can't dress like a lady, because then people would think I wasn't serious, that I cared too much about clothes. I can't wear anything that looks as if too much thought went into it."

She invests in clothes that are well-made, well-cut and of high quality. But they are never fussy or flamboyant. "I can wear things that are gorgeous by themselves, but I can't wear anything fussy. Knits are terrific because they look fancy and serious and ladylike without having that corporate look. Suits can be wonderful but if you don't do them right, they can turn yuppie on you. A great suit looks very serious but not very journalistic. A jacket, unless it's soft, is probably not good because it's too hard. It's too encasing, too closed. Knits can have a little more imagination. They look a little less like something an authority figure would wear. So they're better for doing an interview."

Suzanne Garment is a sophisticated observer of the American scene. She has thought a lot about the way a successful reporter wants to look. "You want to look serious, generally respected, really interested. People tell you things when you look really interested. If you're dressed up too much, they won't talk as openly."

Chapter VII shows how you can build a wardrobe that sets off your unique Communicator profile.

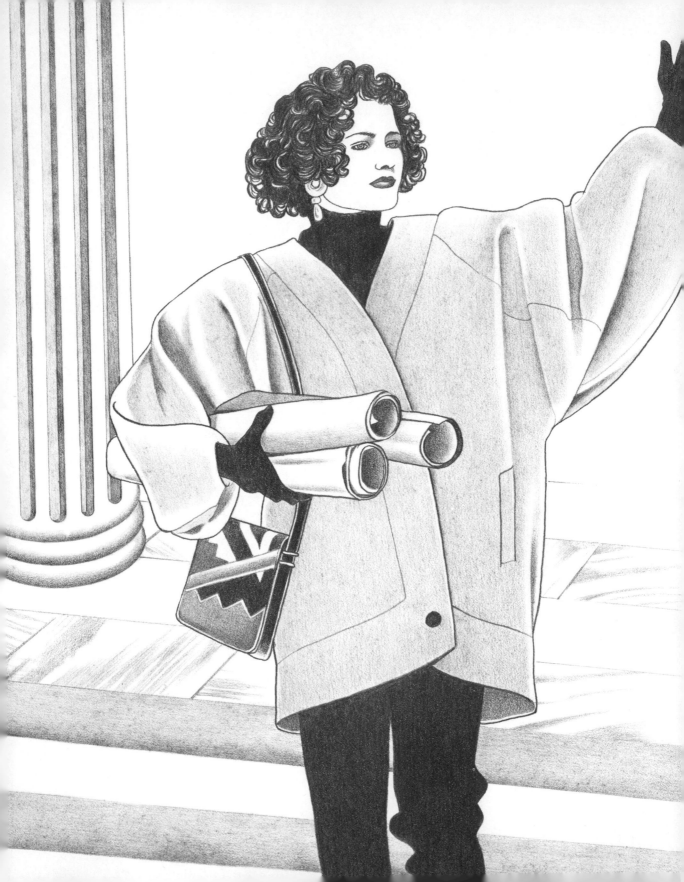

The Creative Profile

The Creative profile is not just for the woman who works in a creative field. It is also for the Corporate and Communicator woman who would like a leisure wardrobe that allows her more imagination. And it is for the woman who travels and would like to pack six suitcases of ideas into one overnight bag. The Creative profile will work for any woman who feels awkward when she enters the world of creative people: the banker who feels out of place in an art gallery; the businesswoman who'd like to change her look when going out with friends after work; the lawyer who has creative clients and feels stuffy around them. This chapter is about what a woman can do to create her own look. It shows you how almost any woman can develop a more creative eye and have an individual style and flair.

"Creative" encompasses far more than the fields of the arts. There are creative jobs, creative companies and creative people in many parts of the business world. It's not uncommon, for example, to find a situation in a single company where there's a split down the middle: the serious, corporate world on one side; the imaginative, creative world on the other. The woman who feels restrained and restricted by the corporate structure should be aware that there is plenty of room in the working world for the more experimental, freewheeling creative personality. In fields such as advertising, retailing, fashion, cosmetics and interior design, as well as areas connected to the theater, television, the performing arts, painting, sculpture, music and writing, women are exploring and developing career opportunities. In jobs that range from editors and copy writers to clothing designers and photographers, from producers and publicists to museum curators and gallery coordinators, the creative career possibilities are ever-increasing.

The Creative person, no matter what her job, is most concerned with her own accomplishments. She doesn't reach upward like the Corporate person, doing the job well so that she can climb the ladder of success. Nor does she reach outward for success, like the Communicator, by developing relationships with people outside the organization. The Creative individual looks inward for gratification and career achievement. That is not to say that material rewards do not count, or that promotions are unimportant. They do count and they are important, but they come from success in reaching inward.

It is the ability to be innovative, imaginative and inventive that distinguishes the Creative profile. The Creative person must feel relaxed and unrestrained in the way she dresses. But in the career world, she must be conscious of the impact of her appearance on colleagues, clients and critics. Because she often sells her talent to new clients, she must be able to express her imagination in her appearance. It's particularly important that the Creative person be aware of other people's need to perceive her as talented. They have certain expectations of how she should look. Those expectations may combine an artistic flair with some identification with themselves. A woman who exudes self-confidence, individuality, and a sharp eye for color, texture and form, is conveying her creative ability.

More than any other group, the Creative woman must dress to please herself and to express her personality. She is her most important audience. Whether she is decked out in designer clothes, thrift shop finds or Minimalist pieces, she is making a statement about herself and her talents. Her success depends on her ability to produce imaginatively, inventively and with originality.

The Creative profile covers a number of different fields: in the world of fashion and cosmetics, it relates to stylists and designers; in fashion retailing, it encompasses fashion buyers and coordinators and the creative support talent of a store—everyone from the display team to publicity and special events managers; in the world of home furnishings, it includes designers and decorators; in newspapers and magazines, editors and photographers; in radio and television, directors and producers; and in museums and art galleries, curators, publicists, and the artists themselves.

All of these positions are linked by an aesthetic appreciation. The Creative profile is underlined by a sensitivity to colors, to shape and to texture. What better place to express this sensitivity than in one's own appearance. The way a woman puts herself together suggests how she will put other things together, how imaginative her product will be.

This artistic flair doesn't necessarily mean complex dressing, nor need it be outrageous. It can range from contemporary to avant-garde, although sometimes it's expressed best through spareness. Purity of line and form can be as complete as a multi-layered outfit. Artistic flair can be registered through use of a single color, an outstanding accessory, or anything else that helps to define your uniqueness. For example, fashion authority Diana Vreeland is known for her dramatic approach. As a reaffirmation of that, her favorite color is clear, strong red. She uses it in her lipstick, on her nails and in her clothes. Similarly Paloma Picasso, a successful designer in her own right and daughter of the artist Pablo Picasso, wears pale makeup and strong red lipstick. On another color wave, the artist Louise Nevelson, known for her rather mysterious black constructions, always appears shrouded in layers of black clothing.

Most important of all, these women have a strong sense of themselves. They know what they like and what looks best on them. That means they may not always follow what's in fashion. In actuality, the truly Creative woman makes her own fashion. She also has a precision, a character, in her appearance that says she cares about herself and about her work.

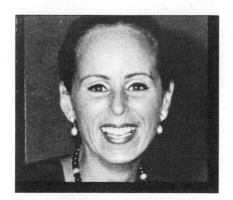

ALYCE FINELL: PRODUCER

Alyce Finell has been involved with the arts in one way or another since she was a young girl. Her first ambition was to become a musician. Later on she moved into the world of television, where she worked as a writer and producer, and today she is responsible for programming for a large cable network. Finell also produces off-Broadway plays and full-length films.

You know when you see her that she is bright, energetic and imaginative. For one thing, it's hard to imagine Finell without a hat. It has become her trademark, and her signal to the world that she is an unusual woman. She wears solid colors which are dramatic, and big, bold accessories.

She says she wants to be perceived as "a person who is finished, who has a sense of herself which is personified in dress. I want them to see a secure person, who is maybe a touch different than everybody else. I want to show individuality."

Because she is constantly wrestling with her weight, she must use her creative ingenuity to find clothes that will give her a clean, clear line. "I have to apply every trick of the trade to hide my flaws," she openly admits. She avoids wearing prints, and stays with solid colors in neutrals, such as beige or khaki, or black.

"I always have something available in black," she says. She may wear it alone or bring in a bold color accent. "I like a shock of color. Sometimes I'll wear black with bright blue, black with purple, or black with hot pink."

She wears stockings in the color of her shoes or the color of her dress to give her a longer, leaner look. She also uses bold accessories and bows at the neck. Like her hats, they draw attention to her face and away from her figure. They also give her a more dramatic look. And for a woman on any kind of budget, accessories change the look of the dress. "They can take a nothing-looking dress and make it something special," she notes. When she buys jewelry, she likes big pieces. A favorite brass pendant, designed by Yves St. Laurent, finishes off many different outfits. Finell changes the silk cord it hangs on to coordinate with the different colors of her clothes.

Finell enjoys clothes and doesn't let her figure problems spoil her fun. With her vivid imagination and sharp color sense, she turns dressing into an adventure. She presents a striking picture wherever she goes and sends a message that she is a Creative woman.

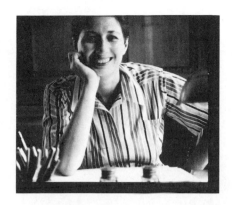

Rachel Newman is editor-in-chief of *Country Living* magazine. Her career in the magazine world has taken her from fashion to home furnishings. In both fields she is very aware of how people look. She says, "I watch what people are wearing. I have to say that I frequently make decisions about people, in terms of the job, depending upon how they put themselves together." She is quick to point out that expensive clothes are not the answer. To her, successful dressing means imagination and style. "I don't think that has to mean how they've done it financially, or anything else, but actually how they've put the outfits together."

When Newman is hiring people for her staff, her goal is to seek people who are innovative. "For the magazine, I essentially feel they have to be creative people generally. Taste and flair go from one area to the next. You can generally tell by the way somebody is putting themselves together how they'll react in a room or on a set."

It is more than just coordinating an outfit that is important, however. Like the successful Corporate woman or Communicator, the Creative person should be precise. Newman adds, "The other thing that I think is very important is the line, the basic line, and whether the person is neat and clean. I know that sounds very old-fashioned, but that is very important to me, because that says something else. To me it says something about their organization and whether or not they keep their business life in order as well."

Even though her background is in fashion, Newman does not give fashion the highest priority. She says, "I don't care if the person is not the most forward in terms of fashion. The other element, the idea of being an individual, is very important to me in terms of this magazine. I want people to have opinions and a sense of themselves. If they dress in their own personal style, I think that's wonderful. I respond to an attempt to create a personal style."

Unlike the corporate world, where the team uniform is relatively similar, there is no single style that predominates in the Creative profile. As one woman on Newman's staff put it, "Magazines can be a little risky and all-embracing. There isn't a code. I think if some of the people went to Wall Street they wouldn't even be hired." Newman adds, "The suit look with the floppy tie—that really wouldn't get by in our industry. Somebody who wears that every day, to me, is someone who has absolutely no imagination, no creativity. It's such a cliché on the streets of New York now. At the magazine, for example, in the spirit of individuality, each woman is encouraged to develop her own look."

Yet in the very same company, on the business side, the approach is the opposite. "On the advertising side, it's not that way. You'll see a lot of suits over there." Newman attributes this to their audience. "They're much more into the male world. They speak to men."

Rachel Newman's audience is diverse. She may be traveling, which she often does, visiting furniture manufacturers or readers' homes to be photographed for the magazine. She may be working in New York with designers. Or she may be meeting in her own offices with the magazine's business staff. No matter whom she is working with, Newman says, "I've always been drawn to colors. I've always liked quality and I could never afford what I wanted, so I bought all my clothes on sale. No one else wanted it. I wanted the offbeat colors." She knows there are looks she can wear around her editorial office that would not work across the hall, so she adapts and adjusts her style slightly. A favorite pair of bold parrot shaped earrings are lots of fun. She says, "Around here people love them. But I know, if I ever wore those earrings into an advertising business meeting, it would be awful."

Like most women, her style has evolved, changing with her job, her taste and her figure. "My lifestyle seems to be traveling. I've gotten away from the classic tailored suits. I don't think I look as good in them since I've put on weight. I'm now wearing a lot of knits, with basic lines as much as possible. I'm at the point where I don't want miscellaneous items around my closet. I'm not interested in buying unless it's a very, very basic kind of thing. Knits do the job for me." Lately, Newman has favored knit dresses from Adrienne Vittadini. For a two week vacation in Europe, she took just two simple Vittadini dresses, one in black and one in red, changed them each day, and sparked them up with witty accessories such as star-shaped pavé "diamond" earrings or her colorful parrot ones.

As for her image and the way she wants her audience to see her, Newman says, "I don't want them to look at me and say that I'm really up-to-date with my clothes. I want them to say that my clothes look good on me."

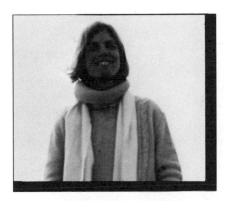

B O   N I L E S :
E D I T O R

The creative process means constantly learning and adapting. One of the people Newman emulates is Bo Niles, senior editor on the magazine. Niles worked for *Mademoiselle* for several years before joining *Country Living*. She notes with satisfaction that even high profile fashion editors prefer quality to quantity and individuality to following any fads. She says, "When I was working at *Mademoiselle,* the highest level fashion editors had the fewest clothes. They were so secure in their image. What they chose was the consummate in quality. They always had the best cashmere or the best wool and the best tailored clothes. They might not necessarily always buy the most expensive designer, but dressing was done with such precision and care that they could repeat the clothes daily with just a few accessories and exude confidence."

Although their clothes are simple, Niles points out that they are neither boring nor brash. "Even though they're confident and composed, they're willing to take that one little risk. They're making a statement of their own look through their clothing, but it's compatible with the job they're in. They're not going to do something flamboyant or flashy or grotesque. They're conscious of what they are and what their job is. It comes across as complete. It doesn't have to be tailored into a stereotype." Niles prefers perfectly simple, spare clothes: She might wear a crisp, cream-colored cotton sleeveless sweater over a long, easy, beige linen skirt, or a pared-down V-neck dress that emphasizes pure line and color.

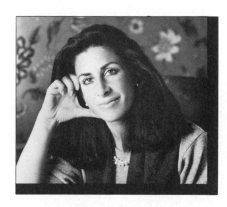

LYNN ROBERTS:
FASHION
EXECUTIVE

Fashion is business but dressing is fun for Lynn Roberts, director of advertising and public relations for the Echo Design Group. In her position she works with people on both the business and creative side of fashion: buyers and top management of department stores like Macy's and Bloomingdale's; fashion editors from major magazines; her firm's public relations and advertising agencies. She may spend one day in her office, another in the showroom, and yet another at outside meetings or on location for a photography shoot. Roberts says, "I think because I'm involved in sales I want to dress fashionably but not too kooky. On the other hand, I want to be businesslike. I think anyone who's selling fashion should project it. What's fun about being in this business is that you can get away with wearing almost anything. I do think about who I'm working with that day and how I want to look. If I'm meeting store executives, I want to look businesslike. If I'm meeting advertising people, I can wear blue jeans."

On the day we met she wore a long, white varsity sweater, a $2 T-shirt which she bought in a variety store, a long, navy pleated skirt, white knee socks and tasseled loafers. "I change my look all the time," she says. "Today I look schoolgirl. Tomorrow I might wear pants and an oversized sweater and the next day a suit."

Whatever she wears, there is always attention to details, a twist of interesting textures, and good mix of colors. Says Roberts, "I like things that are unusual. I like novelty fabrications. I love interesting sweaters. I love dark colors—black, navy, charcoal, brown and green with touches of red. I like mixing patterns and textures together. A friend who is a lawyer saw me one day with different things and said, 'How did you put that all together? I could never do it.' I was wearing tweed pants, a plaid shirt, and a patterned sweater."

Roberts has developed her Creative eye over the years. Of course, she is exposed to a continuous supply of fresh ideas from the fashion industry itself. Nevertheless, that too can be overwhelming and confusing. She experiments to see what looks best on her, then has the self-assurance to adapt a style and carry it through. She says, "I think you have to trust yourself and have the confidence that you can make it work for you."

FAYE LANDAU: FASHION RETAILER

Another woman who has spent many years in the fashion business is Faye Landau. One of the few but growing number of women in top management, she was a vice president of a major west coast department store chain before establishing her own business.

Landau compares herself to friends who dress for the corporate world and says, "I have a strong aversion to what I deem the IBM suit. In my business you don't want to dress like that. You want to be fashion-aware." She makes a distinction between knowledge and application. "You don't have to be fashion forward, but you have to know what's going on: the right color combinations, the right fabrics, when you do wear pants, when you don't wear pants, and when you wear pants, the right pants."

Women who work in the fashion business have an audience of fashion experts. In that sense they must conform to the fashion language, often dressing in recognizable designer clothes, yet giving their appearance a look of individuality. Their job is to keep abreast of the newest directions and set the tone for others in the store and for customers. They must be aware of the trends and adapt them to their own style to signal their creativity. The team uniform becomes their adaptation of the latest fashion looks.

Landau says, "No one ever said I was expected to look the part. I got hired for my talent but there was also no question that I was asked to conform. You knew you were expected to because everyone else did."

Nevertheless, Landau enjoyed the experimental environment, the challenge of the change, and the fresh, new ideas that were always emerging. She says, "The top management people definitely had a flair. It was an atmosphere that allowed you to be yourself, allowed you to play. You didn't have to be the same person on Monday and Tuesday and Wednesday and Thursday and Friday. I loved it. I could be preppy on Monday and hot Kamali on Wednesday."

But she never kidded herself into thinking this was only play. Landau knew that what she wore, and how she wore it, had a decided effect on her audience of retailing experts. She was also aware that her clothes signaled how she felt about herself. "I knew that what I wore was going to tell them something about myself throughout the day. There were times when I woke up in the morning and I thought to myself, 'I can hardly pull myself out of bed.' Usually on those days I was very conservative, very preppy, very withdrawn, and I acted that way. On other days I would get up and I had Kamali to the teeth." Whatever the look, Landau gave the clothes her own stamp. There is little respect in the fashion business for people who wrap themselves in designer labels for security. The Creative message comes in the self-confidence of putting the pieces together with ingenuity and panache.

At meetings where Landau presented the ideas of her special events area (a department with a $50 million budget), "authority and confidence" were the power images she wanted to project. To get that message across, she used her creativity to dress the part. She wore neutral colors, nothing bizarre. "I did not wear really strange, hot combinations to those meetings. I wore gorgeous fabrics but the basic style was neutral, so they would listen to me and not pay attention to what I was wearing. I chose the colors I wore and the accessories with a great deal of care."

The styles and shades she selected emphasized her appreciation of quality, as well as her artistic sense of color, line and texture. She wanted to appear authoritative, but never lost track of her identity as a woman. "I tried to pick up colors to give me some sense of femininity. I never wanted to be drab and bland. On the other hand, there was a sense of quiet authority in the clothes I wore." One favorite outfit is a bone-colored silk suit but it is not a traditional suit. The loose jacket is in a wrap style, has wide roll-up sleeves, and is shaped into a point in the back. With it she might choose a turquoise silk blouse, brown shoes and brown handbag, or for a different mood, a cranberry knit top with pink pearls and cranberry shoes. The strong color in the blouse or sweater emphasizes her sociability. The unusual color combination underlines her inventiveness and flair.

The Creative woman may sometimes find herself in the role of a Communicator. When she made her presentations, Landau says, "I was selling concepts, ideas: this is what I think we should do, this is what we should spend. So I needed to make sure that number one, I was comfortable, and number two, that they would be comfortable."

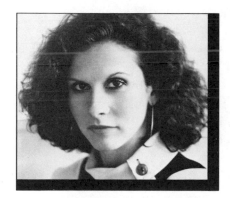

MARIANNE DIORIO: COSMETICS EXECUTIVE

Marianne Diorio, publicity director for Prescriptives cosmetics in New York, has a style that is slightly outrageous. She carries it off with great flair because she believes in her own look. She too worked as a magazine editor before going with her present job. She says she has toned down her look to adapt to the more conservative world of cosmetics. Although her style is still fanciful, it is compatible with the image of her company.

Although many Corporate women have little time or interest in shopping, the Creative woman finds it another outlet for ideas. Diorio enjoys shopping, picking up different looks from dime stores as well as elegant boutiques. "I am a very democratic shopper. I shop everywhere from Lamston's to Bendel's," she says.

Her audience is primarily the beauty editors of newspapers and magazines. She also works with photographers and others who are creative resources for the company. These are the people she sees all the time. As professionals in the fashion and beauty business, they appreciate, if not expect, Creative dressing. But Diorio also works with people on the business side of her organization. She dresses accordingly, and says, "At sales meetings I can't look like a total freak or else no one will take me seriously. I might tend to be a little more conservative than if I were having lunch with the editor from *Self.* So it depends within a certain realm. But I've never been very conservative, and I've never worn anything very conservative."

The day we met she was dressed in a turquoise oversized jacket designed by Cathy Hardwick, a purple sweater that she had kept from her high school days, a black skirt, black stockings and pink shoes which she had bought in Italy. That may sound like a mishmash, but—with her terrific eye for color and shape—Diorio had pulled it together and looked great. At the same time, she was making a fashion statement for her company, reinforcing its young, aggressive, upscale image.

Diorio says, "Fashion has an influence. If we say people are wearing neon colors, or black with a shock of pink, it's important that I follow through in that statement with what I wear. Usually it's something that I'd buy anyway, so I'm not compromising myself. It's important also that the editors perceive of Prescriptives as very modern and up-to-date. Since I'm the spokesperson for that company, it's important for me to look that way and be that way."

There are several things she takes into account when she is getting dressed: whom she's meeting, the image of her company, and how she wants to be perceived. Diorio says, "I want people to think I'm creative but in control; that I'm full of ideas but a real person." When *Cosmopolitan* magazine interviewed her about the way she dresses, she told them, "I'm not one of those women who'd wear pinstripe suits and those little ties. I want to look finished, yet I want to look creative." She explains how her look might change from day to day as she tries out new styles, new ways of dressing, keeping her agenda in mind. "There are some days I'll walk in and I'll have on a big blue parachute linen outfit with neon orange stockings. The next day I might wear a suit. It depends on the occasion too."

Is the inventive Diorio always confident, or does she ever put an outfit together and then wonder what she has done? "Yes," she answers, "a lot. But I think you have to take that risk. Take a chance. I live through it. . . . Who cares if someone doesn't like it? If they don't like it, too bad." But her dressing is never haphazard. She cares about her look, tests new styles, and pays great attention to how she puts the pieces together to achieve a complete look. "I would say that there has to be a certain sense that a person has put some thought into how to make it work even if it's bizarre. That gives it a finished look. It's *premeditated creativity*. I think a woman has to take time with her clothes, try them on, and have an experimenting session with herself." Diorio may find dressing amusing, but she takes her appearance seriously.

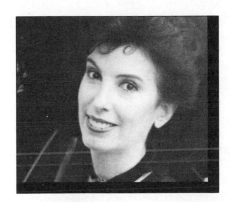

DENA SOLLINS: ARTS CONSULTANT

Far from the world of fashion and cosmetics, another career woman, Dena Sollins, has spent most of her time working with artists. For many years she has done interviews for National Public Radio and the Canadian Broadcasting Company. She has also coordinated arts projects for major corporations and helped to start a women's museum. In her different roles, she has experimented with various styles of dressing from designer suits to decidedly hippie looks. With her pale skin and auburn hair, she favors strong colors or pale ivories, and always adapts them into dramatic styles. The day we met she was dressed in an ivory silk tunic dress printed with splashes of brilliant poppies. With it she wore a big brimmed poppy-colored hat.

Because she is so conscious of the effect of clothing on artistic sensibilities, she is careful to dress differently for each person she interviews. But she always dresses with imagination. Like Landau, there are times when she is in the Communicator role, and she adapts her Creative style to it. Says Sollins, "If I'm interviewing Eudora Welty, for example, I'm not going to dress like a young, hip kid. I'll dress in something that makes her feel comfortable when we sit down. When she first sees me, she is not going to think, 'Oh my, look at this person. How much does she know about my writing? Look at the age difference.' As an interviewer, you're really a tool to bring the other person out. My personality should not be an intrusion into the interview. If I'm interviewing a person who's younger than I am, I won't wear a suit. It depends on the subject of the interview. I think it's especially important in an interview, if you're trying to bring the other person out and get information, that they're in no way stymied or inhibited by something that's exterior like your clothing. If I'm interviewing Bob Rauchenberg I will dress very differently. Whatever instills confidence and makes somebody comfortable I do."

She has found that the way she dresses has a definite impact on her mood and her abilities. She says, "I think suits look terrific on many women. They suit the suit. But my personality is limited by suits. When I close the button on the jacket, especially on a very tailored conservative suit, I just find it's much more difficult to express my self. I think it affects my personality. I become subdued and my behavior is more controlled."

Creative dressing can mean a marked style that is always yours or it can mean a different look every day. It always includes originality and, as Marianne Diorio put it, premeditation, because creative dressers enjoy the most latitude in what they may wear. Rarely does a woman who dresses creatively just throw her clothes on and run out the door. If she does, she probably thought about them the night before. Like most artists, creative dressers learn from others. They watch, test and try to see what will work for them. You can get ideas from all sorts of sources: in museums looking at paintings; walking down the street and watching other women; in newspapers, magazines and books. But the creative part comes in the privacy of your own bedroom, where you can take those ideas and try them with your own clothes. It may be a matter of adding a scarf to your dress and then tying it a new way, or belting a jacket and lifting the collar, or mixing the colors in an outfit for a new combination. The more you try, the more you learn, and the stronger the message will be that you too are a Creative woman.

How's Your Capsule Concept?

Try this quiz to see how well planned your wardrobe is.

1. When you look in your closet do you see:

a) A lot of clothes and nothing to wear ☐
b) A few things you like and a lot you never wear ☐
c) A few well-loved items which go with nothing ☐
d) Several good items which work together ☐

2. Are your clothes in colors that:

a) Look like everything in the rainbow ☐
b) Sometimes go together ☐
c) Were all the rage last year ☐
d) Coordinate well with each other ☐

3. Do you have:

a) A lot of clothes in the same style ☐
b) A lot of clothes that are boring ☐
c) Styles which you wore in school ☐
d) A variety of styles to choose from ☐

4. If someone calls you at the last minute to go out to lunch, do you:

a) Feel like hiding under your desk ☐
b) Say ok but wish you had worn something else ☐
c) Say yes for next week, then go out shopping ☐
d) Say yes immediately because you look great ☐

5. When you look at yourself in the mirror, do you:

a) Look like you wished you worked in a different field ☐
b) Look like you wished you worked for a different company ☐
c) Look like you're still in school ☐
d) Look like the image of your company and your field ☐

6. Do you:

a) Never try new combinations with your clothes ☐
b) Once in a while try to put things together ☐
c) Wear your outfits exactly as you bought them ☐
d) Always experiment with new combinations ☐

7. Do you wish you could:

a) Throw out everything and start again ☐
b) Buy a lot of new clothes ☐
c) Buy one new item to update your clothes ☐
d) Buy a few new things to perk up your wardrobe ☐

8. Do people in your organization:

a) Hint that you are dressed inappropriately ☐
b) Say you look nice about twice a year ☐
c) Say they would like to dress like you ☐
d) Admire your originality ☐

9. When you get dressed in the morning do you:

a) Try on lots of outfits ☐
b) Grab the tried, the true ☐
c) Experiment, but feel uncomfortable half the time ☐
d) Know whatever you put on will look good ☐

10. When you are getting dressed do you:

a) Never have the right shoes ☐
b) Always change your handbag to match your clothes ☐
c) Look pretty good but find you are always missing one accessory ☐
d) Look really coordinated ☐

Score 1 point for each "a"; 3 points for each "b"; 5 points for each "c"; 7 points for each "d". EVALUATION: *9 points—Read this book again; 10–27—Your wardrobe needs some more work; 28–45—Keep trying, you're on the right track; 46–70—You're doing great.*

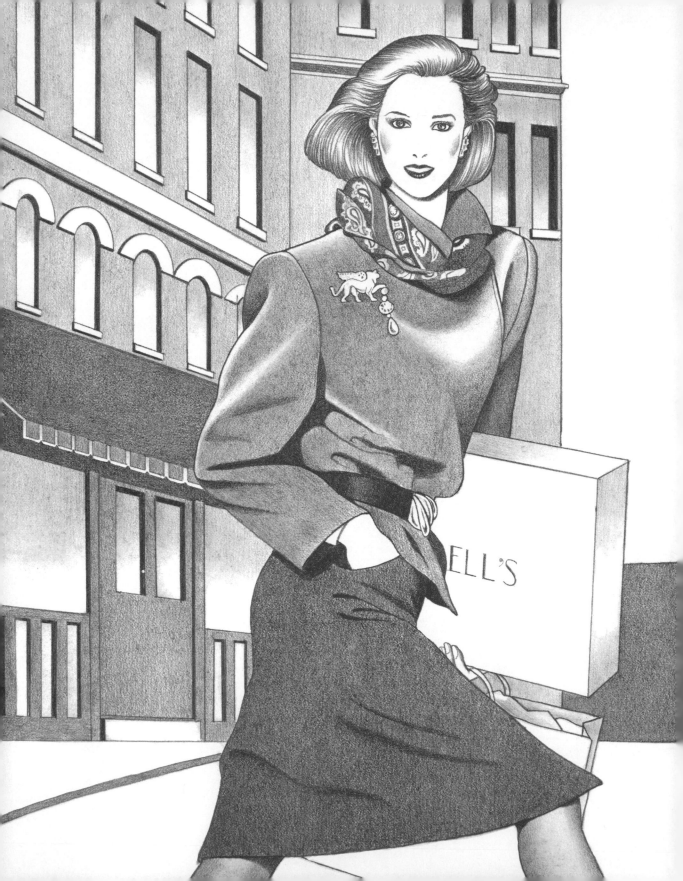

CHAPTER V

Building Your Wardrobe

P art of the trick of building a successful wardrobe is in choosing styles that are classics, that transcend time. Classic refers to fine fabrics, well-cut styles, good fit and traditional colors. A prime example is the classic designs of Coco Chanel, clothes that are still elegant more than fifty years after she created them. Today, along with the designs from Chanel, the styles of Yves Saint Laurent, Calvin Klein, Ralph Lauren and Bill Blass combine high-quality fabrics and well-

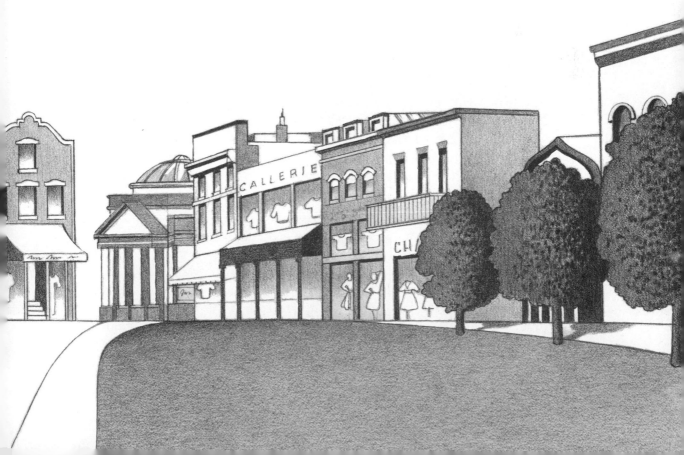

cut, classic lines with contemporary touches. These kinds of clothes signal your interest in good quality, whether in your wardrobe or in your work. Even at less expensive price points, you can find clothes with the cut and flair that express your interest in the best.

The most attractively dressed women often combine their classic clothes with touches of individuality, and their ideas may come from the fashion trends for the season. For instance, a navy suit can be updated with colorful jewelry one year, a big scarf the next, and have a pared-down look the next. But whatever is in fashion, the most successful personal style is one which allows you to feel self-confident without being self-conscious.

The role of fashion can sometimes be confusing: Clothes may look wonderful in magazines, or be attractive in the stores, but they may not seem applicable to your own lifestyle. Fashion, however, is a part of the times and keeping up with it is part of being in tempo, like seeing the latest movies, reading the latest books, or trying the newest trends in food. Finding just what suits you best, from all the choices that are available, is a weeding-out process; there may be only one or two ideas you like, but finding them is worth the effort.

For most of us, the high-fashion look that says "dressed to kill" is too threatening. It doesn't belong in the Corporate or Communicator arena unless you're part of the fashion world, and even then it must be used carefully or it will be too intimidating. Yet applying some of these ideas can be a way of refreshing your perspective. The ideal wardrobe for most working women, whether Corporate, Communicator or Creative, is one which includes classic looks and contemporary touches.

When the editors of *Vogue* magazine organized a symposium of high-powered women, the subject was fashion and working women. Included in the group were Dianne Feinstein, Mayor of San Francisco; Mary Wells Lawrence, chairman of Wells, Rich, Greene; and Brenda Landry, vice president, Morgan Stanley. Each talked about how her wardrobe is adapted to her career needs.

As an officer of a major financial institution, Brenda Landry is a Corporate woman. She describes being invited to address a group of top male and female MBA students from around the United States. All of the people in the audience were dressed in the standard navy and gray. She says, "I had on my typical 'uniform', something conservative— a red Adolfo suit, pearls, a pair of slingback shoes." The women students came up to Landry afterwards to find out if they really didn't have to dress in gray flannel blazers and low-heeled shoes. She says, "I think it is detrimental to your career to come in for a job interview dressed like that . . . if you're looking for high-powered talent you are not looking for somebody who is pedestrian. Clothing, fashion, makeup, accessories, fragrance: They're all part of the stage of life. If you don't care, you stay in the back row in your uniform."

Women who are successful know how to use clothing as a tool. Mary Wells Lawrence, chairman of a large advertising agency and the woman who gained fame putting Pucci designs on airline stewardesses says, "I have always used fashion in my business life to create an image and an atmosphere that are comfortable. . . . Fashion can make others comfortable or uncomfortable and should be looked at in that way. The way you look is the first thing a person knows about you, the first signal of what you're like. The impression you make can say you're going to make someone nervous, you're going to be too chic, you're going to be too masculine, you're going to be too hostile . . . I have always chosen business clothes from Yves Saint Laurent, because he does classic things. I use Chanel . . . for classic suits that make me look like a put-together lady: neat, not threatening and yet, at the same time, smart. That's what Saint Laurent's classics and Chanel's things convey. That's quite different from looking unfashionable."

As Mayor of San Francisco, Dianne Feinstein is always in the public eye. She represents a major American city and addresses a large and varied audience. She wears tailored suits and soft blouses to achieve a look that is crisp, neat and affable from early morning to late at night.

THE CAPSULE CONCEPT

Building an effective wardrobe requires time and thought, not to mention money. That is why I have developed the Capsule Concept, an easy, efficient way to have a small wardrobe that stretches to a great number of different looks. A "Capsule" is a small group of clothes, preferably about twelve pieces, based around two colors, with all the pieces working together. This means that your jackets can be worn with all of your skirts, pants and dresses; your blouses can be worn with all of your skirts and pants (and even with some of your dresses); and your skirts, pants and dresses will go with all of your tops. With this interchangeability, a small group of twelve pieces can be extended to make as many as forty different outfits.

For the past several years I've held seminars and fashion shows in department stores around the country from New York to Los Angeles, Dallas to Detroit and many points in between. One of the most exciting things for me has been to see how Capsules can be made with many different kinds of clothing for many different types of people and different lifestyles. I've selected styles from high-priced designer boutiques to low-priced budget areas, from advanced fashion looks to solidly conservative styles. I've used dark colors such as navy, wine, black and gray; dark and light combinations such as navy and beige, or black and white; and even included brights such as purple and red, or turquoise and pink. I've created Capsules using moderate-priced clothing from manufacturers such as Chaus and Koret, or better-priced clothing from firms such as Liz Claiborne and Evan Picone, or from designers such as Calvin Klein and Yves Saint Laurent.

You can do this too. You read about the three different profiles: Corporate, Communicator and Creative. The following chapters show you how these profiles can be interpreted into Capsules. You'll also learn how you can let your own personality come through so that your Capsule reflects your individuality.

Keep in mind that most women don't have to go out and purchase a whole new wardrobe to fit their Capsule profile. Most of us have some of the pieces already in our closet. It may not seem that way now. As you look at your clothes you may feel a hopeless sense of confusion. It may look as though nothing goes with anything else. But don't despair. As you begin to rethink your approach to dressing, you'll see that many of the components in your closet can work in different ways. For example, skirts that are part of suits can be worn with different jackets and different tops. Jackets that seem to go only with the skirt they came with may actually look better with different skirts or dresses. You'll see how to put colors together that you never thought would work together, and you'll learn how those new combinations can update your wardrobe.

Begin to create your Capsule with the clothes in your own closet. Take the clothes you have and hang them by color, going from light to dark. Include your dresses, skirts, pants and jackets so that you hang all of one color together. That is, put all of your navy clothes together, all of your wine clothes together and so on. You'll begin to see that there are probably two or three colors that predominate. These colors can be the basis of your Capsule. If you have some clothes that are in prints or patterns, such as a favorite plaid jacket or print skirt, you may want to choose from these colors to form your Capsule.

You may find you have at least the beginnings of one or two Capsules in your closet. For example, you may own one gray suit which you really like, or you may have a few separates, such as skirts and jackets, in navy and wine, that seem to all work together. Even if you would like to discard most of your clothes, if you have just one jacket or skirt or dress that you like, that component can become the beginning of a Capsule.

After you've decided on the colors for your Capsule, try on the different pieces in that group and see how they work together. Separate the jackets and skirts of your suits so that they become individual pieces and not just part of a suit. Hang them separately in your closet so that you'll begin to think of them not just as a single outfit but as components of your Capsule. As you go through this book, you'll see many ideas for forming Capsule combinations. Some of these may be combinations that you never thought would work together. You'll be surprised and pleased to learn that there is great hidden potential for your Capsule wardrobe right in your closet. With the right basic pieces, you can develop a wardrobe strategy that allows you to go from a conservative Corporate profile to an innovative Creative profile.

Remember too that as your audience changes, your profile may change; you may be a Corporate woman at one point, a Communicator at another, and a Creative at the next. By knowing how to adjust your wardrobe to these different needs, you can add to its power. The basic navy dress exemplifies this point. It's the type of dress that can be in any woman's wardrobe and can be adjusted for different situations. When worn with the matching navy jacket, it becomes an authoritative outfit for the Corporate woman. Worn alone, it speaks well for the Communicator as a finished, yet not constricting outfit. And when the same dress is worn with a sweater underneath or a vest on top, there is an added element of innovation and a relaxed attitude that is appropriate for the Creative woman. This dress can also be adapted for the evening by adding jewelry.

As you put together the components in your Capsule, keep in mind that each piece of clothing has its own message. In a sense, each component is like a phrase in a sentence. When you combine the phrases, you are forming a strong visual message. A constructed jacket is authoritative; a blouson jacket is casual; a straight skirt is direct; a pair of skinny pants is sexy; a ruffled blouse is coquettish.

Colors also play an important part in the message: Some colors are more powerful, some are friendlier, some are dressier, some are more casual. When used with certain clothes, the effect may vary from intimidating to innovative. The cardigan jacket is far more authoritative in navy than in hot pink. The blazer may be conservative in charcoal gray, aggressive in fire engine red. When you learn the sorts of signals the components suggest, and what they signify when they are combined, you'll be able to send the message you want known about yourself.

JACKETS. Jackets that are constructed, i.e. have a collar and lapels, set-in sleeves, back seam and lining, take their cue from the styles worn by business and professional men. They suggest power and are particularly useful for the Corporate profile. But these are not the only looks that are appropriate for that category. Jackets that are constructed with straight, clean lines and set-in sleeves may vary from single-breasted lapels to sophisticated cardigans, and each of these expresses authority. The single-breasted jacket, however, which is a copy of a man's jacket, carries a masculine connotation while the cardigan is clearly more refined and ladylike. The woman who wants to be perceived as "one of the boys" might choose the single-breasted version; the woman who wants to suggest more femininity might wear the cardigan. Of course, the same woman may choose to wear the blazer on some occasions and the cardigan on others.

Naturally, not all jackets are as constructed as these. Some have raglan or dolman sleeves which give a less rigid, more relaxed attitude. They work well for the woman who doesn't want to appear intimidating but still wants to add a finished look to her outfit. These less threatening styles can be more effective for a Communicator or Creative woman, who may even resort to the very casual blouson style which is sometimes called a "baseball jacket."

SKIRTS. Skirts that are simple and straight suggest an ordered, neat manner. When straight skirts are eased with pleats or shirring, they suggest a more feminine attitude. Be very aware of the fit, however: Tight skirts send a message that is sexy; the fuller the skirt, the less efficient you can appear. For the woman who wants to suggest crispness, a straight skirt is ideal. The woman who wants to send a message of softness will do better with a fuller style.

A skirt and jacket that are in the same color and fabric, of course, make a matched suit. This combination gives a unified look which signals singular direction. On the other hand, a jacket and skirt that are in different colors suggest diversity. Even though they may be bought together as a suit, they have a less unified look than a matched suit. Accessories or trim may be used to achieve a more coordinated, more integrated look to the outfit.

BLOUSES. Blouse styles also vary and create different effects. Tailored shirt styles with pointed collars and with or without lapels have a clean, efficient look. When the collar is worn closed it suggests a person who is closed up and in control; worn open, the message is more open and relaxed. Jewel neck blouses represent a spare, no frills approach; blouses with bows are softer; ruffles and lace look coy. Very high necklines create an image that is cool and standoffish; very low necklines are sexually inviting.

SWEATERS. Sweaters are always less formal than blouses. They have a more casual look which is often effective for the Communicator or Creative woman, but usually inappropriate for the Corporate Capsule. Cardigan sweaters can be worn in place of a jacket when they have a bulky knit and padded or molded shoulders which lend an air of authority.

DRESSES. In dresses, as in most other clothes, the most classic looks come with simple, clean-lined styles. The most efficient looks are shirtdresses, which take their cue from a man's shirt. The shirtdress can be made more authoritative with the addition of a constructed jacket. Variations on the shirtdress theme, from plain, button-front styles to more sophisticated coatdresses, all have a crisp look that can be appropriate to almost any Capsule. Shifts, or simple, straight-lined dresses, can also suggest a straightforward approach. Fussy designs, however, take the focus away from efficiency. Hemlines above the knee or below the calf are distracting, as are fancy necklines and complicated details.

All of these signals must be combined with the colors of the clothes to complete the message. They may dilute a story or make it strong; unify it or pull it apart. The very nature of the message changes as the colors change. Not only do the colors of an outfit affect its looks—they also affect each other, the wearer and the audience.

COLOR PALETTES

Color theories abound. Women and men all over the country are being color analyzed by color consultants. Whether you seek the advice of a paid consultant or study yourself in the mirror, you will find, quite naturally, that certain colors do look better on you than others. Your skin tone is either warm (yellow) or cool (blue) and the colors you wear will either intensify your features or wash them away. If you haven't already discovered this, then try this experiment. Start with a clean face, no cosmetics, and stand before a mirror with an array of different colors (they may be clothes or scarves that you already own). Hold them up to you, one by one, and see which colors light up your skin, your eyes and your hair. Concentrate on the shades that flatter you, and you can start acquiring more colors in this family. But don't be afraid to experiment.

Color analysis is wonderful if it gives you a positive sense of looking good, but it should not be limiting. There are always new colors coming into fashion, and you would be unfair to yourself if you did not try them. You may find that some of the new shades are not flattering on you; but you will also have the pleasant surprise of discovering colors you may never have thought you could wear. Include those colors in your wardrobe for a contemporary look.

When I was the fashion merchandising director of Garfinckel's, I traveled with our designer buyer to the showrooms in Milan, Paris, London and New York. As we looked at the clothes, we inevitably were attracted to very different colors. Joan is a pale-skinned, platinum blonde who prefers pale, cool colors. I have a more olive complexion and darker hair and favor warm, intense colors. This was a great help in deciding what to buy for the store. We always chose at least two palettes, one for women with cool, pale coloring and one for women with warm, intense coloring. But we would have been foolish not to include new colors each season. By adding at least one new color to your Capsule each season, even if it is in an accessory, you can keep your clothes from being boring or seeming stale.

As you plan your wardrobe, look around at fashion magazines and store displays for new combinations. New color stories appear every season which may freshen up the clothes in your Capsule. You may not even have to buy new clothes to put life in your wardrobe; it may be a matter of rearranging the Capsules you already have. For example, you might have two Capsules in your closet: one in black and gray, the other in red and white. Imagine how different your clothes will look if you recombine them to make two new Capsules, one based on black and white, the other on gray and red.

If you have been color analyzed, you probably have a set of swatches to work with in planning your wardrobe. Use these as a way to begin your Capsules. Take two of your best colors and make them the basis of your Capsule. Then use some of the other colors as accents. But don't neglect new shades that come on the market. I have seen some women reject a color because it isn't on their palette. It is impossible for the consultants to have every imaginable shade in their swatch books. Over and over again, I have shown women new colors to work with that are in their color family.

There are ways of adapting the most flattering shades to your lifestyle. Obviously, if you are a Corporate woman, you may not want to wear pastels all the time. Yet intense colors, such as navy and black, may not always be attractive on you. There are other authoritative shades, such as taupe, beige, and gray, which can be as assertive as the dark ones. There are times, however, when black or navy are the most appropriate colors for the occasion. There are ways to wear them that can still highlight your features; for instance, using the dark colors in your suit, you can wear the more flattering shades close to your face—in your blouse, your scarf or your jewelry. Be aware too, that even black and navy can have warm or cool undertones, and can be dull or bright.

One of the most important things to keep in mind as you combine colors is to be sure to put warm with warm, and cool with cool. A yellow-based (warm) white looks best with yellow-based (warm) black; blue (cool) white looks best with blue (cool) black. As you build your Capsule and experiment with colors, look carefully at the shades to see the undertones. Quite often, in a fashion show or seminar, I will combine pattern with pattern, or color with color, in ways that are out of the ordinary. The audience always admires the clothes, but someone will inevitably ask if it is acceptable to put these looks together. The answer is yes, if you keep to the same cast. This gives a look that is both complementary and harmonious. But the most important point is to use colors that complement you personally and professionally.

COLOR SIGNALS. Patti Mancini is vice president of Rockwell International, the California-based company responsible for the Space Shuttle and other space rockets. Patti is a dynamic redhead who has been with this conservative, male-oriented organization for twenty-three years. As the only woman vice president in the aeronautics industry, she has been influenced more by the male part of the work force than the female. She says, "I think the profession does dictate the appropriate dress. For someone like myself, who's part of a corporation, you pretty much have to abide by their dictates."

You might think that this approach would mean a wardrobe based strictly on suits in navy and gray. But she says, "I always wear suits because my male counterparts wear suits. I like tailored, but not harshly tailored clothes. Where I separate the issue is in colors. I know what colors look good on me, and I tend to stay with them because I feel better then. It's a psychological thing. I don't wear navy pinstripes. I have maintained my individuality. I don't wear peach to the office, but I do wear beiges and taupes. I also have some red suits which I wear." There are times, however, when dark colors are simply more appropriate, especially for a woman who is continuously traveling from her Los Angeles base to Denver, Dallas, New York, Washington, D.C. and Europe. Says Mancini, "I think the situation that you are in dictates what you wear. I do not find that confining. I think you're just more comfortable abiding by that. For instance, black is not a good color on me, but I have some black in my wardrobe because there are times, whatever the event is, that just dictate wearing black or something similar." As for her red suits, "I wear them sometimes giving a speech. I think you need something bright, because it gives you an 'up' feeling. You want to feel 'up' when you're giving a speech." On the other hand, Mancini knows how to use softer shades to make her features stand out. The day we talked she was dressed in a double-breasted, richly textured wool suit in a glen plaid of beige flecked with orange. With it she wore a soft white silk jacquard stock tie blouse, sheer stockings and beige pumps; for jewelry she chose pearl earrings, a gold bracelet and gold rings. Her look was authoritative and feminine. "Women must learn how to use power graciously," she says, and she dresses with the same thought in mind.

Color can be used to enhance your authority or underplay your position. It can send a range of different signals from sincere to sugary, energetic to enervated. Knowing when and how to use color can be critical to your career. If you appear on television or deliver a speech looking washed out, you can lose your audience immediately. If you wear colors that are too aggressive at a meeting where you should blend in, you may damage your position. But if you always blend in, and never stand out, you may disappear into the crowd forever. Karen Valenstein of E. F. Hutton has a range of Chanel-style suits and makes disparaging remarks about young women who look like "little gray mice." She knows when to strike a strong note in navy and when to appear soft in her pastels.

The colors that are most associated with authority are black, navy, gray and beige. But there are other associations with these colors to keep in mind. Several years ago, during a presidential primary campaign, a television network correspondent observed that all of the male

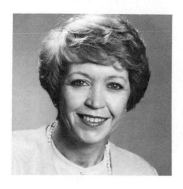 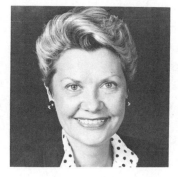

LEFT TO RIGHT:
*Patti Mancini,
Hanne Merriman*

candidates were dressed in navy blue suits. Teamed with the white shirts and red ties that they all wore, the signal was certainly all American red, white and blue. But it also suggested strength in the dark navy, sincerity in the blue, clarity in the white and energy in the red.

Black is used by many women instead of navy. It has the same suggestion of power, though it is slightly more mysterious and can be more flattering to some skin tones. Black is a dressier color than navy, internationally elegant (interestingly, it is the suit color worn in Japan by businessmen and professionals), and because it works well for evening as well as day, black can be an excellent Capsule color for a woman who must make the transition from business to social dressing.

Gray is also a color of strength but with a slightly different tone. "Banker's gray" is an expression that has been used for many years and with good reason. It is a neutral color and connotes a conservative and objective manner, qualities you might look for in a financial manager.

Beige and shades related to it such as tan and taupe have authority and a suggestion of self-containment. Beige is dispassionate and neutral, qualities that are often considered important in the corporate world.

Another color used by corporate women is wine. Although it may suggest less power than the first four colors (perhaps because it is not worn by men), it has other necessary attributes. As a dark member of the red family, wine has authority without being intimidating, energy without being overwhelming.

Brown is a dark color which lacks the power of black, navy, gray or beige, perhaps because of its association with the earth. Rather than the suggestion of sophistication and urbanity which makes the other colors appropriate for the corporate world, brown is connected with rural life. But as Ronald Reagan, the "great communicator," has shown, it can be an effective color to wear.

There are bright colors with great intensity that suggest energy and animation. The strongest of these is red, a color associated with vitality, sexuality and aggression. From the bull fight to the boardroom, red is a dynamic color. Because it has an aura of energy, it is an excellent color for the Communicator. Many women use it when giving a speech or making a television appearance or a presentation.

Other intensely bright colors can also add a burst of energy to your appearance. Some associations with these colors may seem obvious yet make a subtle imprint. Royal blue and purple are rich colors that are associated with royalty. Emerald green expresses new life or regeneration. Gold, of course, is connected to wealth. Shocking pink *is* shocking and hot pink really does make the blood rush. These can be excellent colors when you want to appear vigorous. Although they can be very strong as a total look, taken in small doses, as in blouses or accessories, they can add pep and energy to an otherwise bland outfit.

For many years, Hanne Merriman, the president of Garfinckel's, dressed in shades of gray and beige. Not only were her clothes gray and beige, but her office was gray and beige too. She gave the appearance of a cool, self-confident woman, which was appropriate at the time because she was building a reputation as an effective financial manager for a major chain of stores. After several years of being in the job and wearing this neutral look, a friend convinced her to try a brilliant purple dress. Merriman had established her credibility in the job and could afford to move on to more fashion and vibrancy in her Capsule. The dress drew so many compliments that she began adding more and more vivid colors to her wardrobe. Although she was always well dressed, she had tended towards the conservative end of the fashion spectrum, favoring Calvin Klein over Claude Montana. Even when she wore the newest fashion clothes, they were toned down by the neutral color. The image of the store has been the same: fashion leadership with a refined tone. Once she proved herself, however, she could afford to dress in bolder, stronger colors without risking her reputation as a competent businesswoman. Her image changed from that of an attractively dressed woman to a dynamic fashion leader in her community.

Of course, not everyone can carry off such intense colors. Floral shades such as violet, rose, daffodil and leaf green are slightly less brilliant, yet still bright. These are vibrant enough to add punch but not as overwhelming as the bolder colors. The floral shades can be effective for the Communicator, and in smaller doses, can work well for the Corporate profile.

There is a group of more diluted colors which are sometimes called sherbert shades. These include raspberry, mint, melon, lemon, lime, peach and aqua. For the woman who cannot wear the dynamic colors mentioned above, these shades can be very flattering, particularly in blouses or accessories. Because they lack intensity, they are the opposite of the energetic brights and suggest a milder personality. Although they may not be appropriate in overall dress for the Corporate woman, they can, again, be excellent as accents in accessories or for the Communicator who wants to suggest a soft, unintimidating appearance.

Pastels, such as pink, blue or maize suggest an innocence; these are the colors of the nursery, not usually of the boardroom. But if you know when and how to use them, you can turn them to your advantage.

When Faye Landau was vice president of a major California department store chain, she was asked to attend a meeting with the new head of the store. She knew her boss had heard about her strong personality, and she didn't want him to feel threatened by her. At the meeting she had to make a request for a large increase in her division's multi-million dollar budget. Rather than looking like a sophisticated businesswoman, she wanted to appear soft and even innocent. She decided to wear a pink dress to the meeting, something she had never worn before. The meeting was a success: Her presentation was strong, her personality soft and her budget was increased considerably. Landau has since put the pink dress aside for other emergencies.

The color that best suggests clarity and crispness is white. It is the perfect accompaniment to most suits and an excellent way to pull together skirts and jackets. Like all of the other colors I have mentioned, it can have a cool (blue) cast or a warm (yellow) cast and can include everything from stark white to soft cream.

One time when I was in Philadelphia doing a call-in radio program, a woman called to say that her daughter was having a problem putting together her Capsule. It seems she had bought a gray suit to wear for job interviews and simply could not find the right color blouse to wear with it. When I asked if her daughter had tried white, she said no. She was surprised by the suggestion. I was surprised that she hadn't tried white first. It is the crispest, cleanest color to wear with almost any suit as long as both blouse and suit have the same undertones.

So far I have talked about solid colors. But patterns also send various signals. Solid colors give a look of unity. Although usually not as powerful, some patterns can also be used by the Corporate woman and certainly by the Communicator to express authority. The exception, of course, is pinstripes, which are as powerful as solid colors. Other menswear patterns, such as small checks, tweeds, tattersalls or glen plaids, all have authority. Slightly less intimidating but equally appropriate in the Corporate arena are geometrics, paisleys and foulards.

Naturally, all of these prints work well for the Communicator too, and she can also include florals and plaids. If you wear patterns, keep in mind that the larger the print, the more distracting it becomes. Prints also make an imprint: They are recognizable—by season or by designer—and not as easily changed or disguised as solids. You can have far more versatility in your wardrobe if you concentrate on building Capsules around solid colors and use only a small number of patterns.

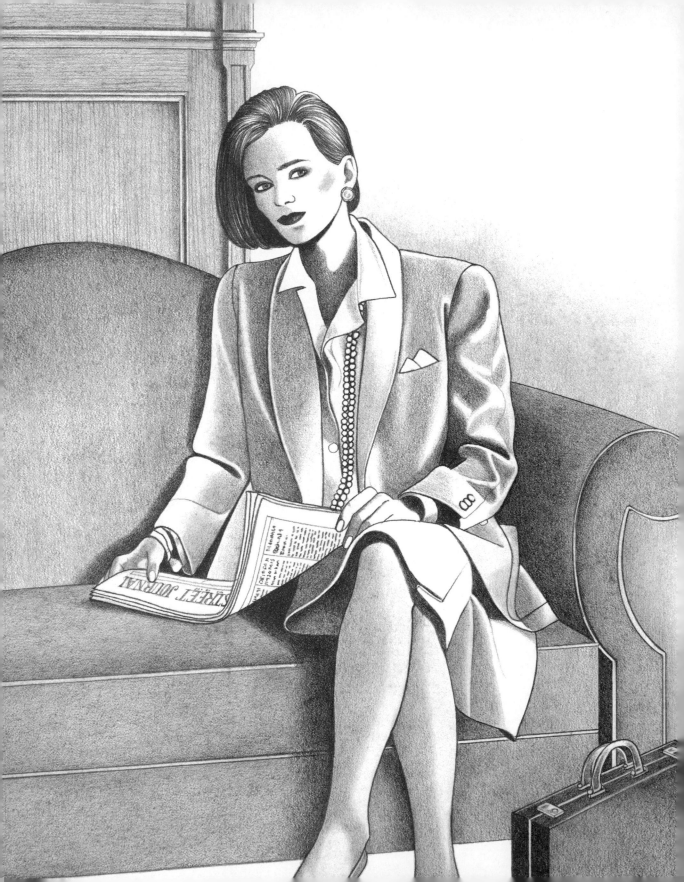

CHAPTER VI

The Corporate Capsule

The Corporate profile is probably the easiest to identify but the most difficult for many women to accept. We all know the male corporate type: the man in the gray flannel suit. In the 1970s women were told that they too had to wear this rigid costume if they were to succeed. Some women jumped on the gray flannel bandwagon and found it successful. Others were repelled by the conformity, the blandness and the loss of female identity.

By now, women have established enough credibility so that there's room in the corporate world not just for gray flannel, but for red silk, pink jersey and a host of other colors and fabrics. The trick is knowing when and where to use them so they add interest without becoming the focal point. The Capsule for the Corporate profile can range from very traditional looks to more contemporary ones. It can include grays and pinks, flannels and jerseys. This chapter presents four Capsules using different color combinations and components so that you can put together a Corporate wardrobe that telegraphs your particular message.

The first Capsule is based on the most traditional profile, appropriate for women starting out in finance or law. It includes solid colors and a minimal number of patterns—i.e. tweeds, checks, stripes, geometrics, paisleys or foulards. There should be at least two matched suits, and the jackets, skirts and dresses should be well-constructed, although there may be knits as well as woven fabrics. The basic colors to choose from are black, navy, gray, brown, beige and wine. Since a Capsule is based around two colors, you have a choice of nine color combinations including black and gray, black and beige, navy and gray, navy and beige, navy and wine, brown and gray, brown and beige, gray and beige, or gray and wine.

THE SUIT. The most important part of the Corporate Capsule is the matched suit. This is the team uniform that speaks the language of the corporate community. The constructed jacket says authority and assertiveness; the tailored skirt suggests femininity and economy; the matched fabric of the jacket and skirt implies organization; the neutral colors underscore seriousness and objectivity.

Look for clothes made in good quality fabrics that are composed of natural fibers. The natural fibers allow the fabric to breathe, so that it is comfortable to wear in all seasons; that is, they keep you warm when it is cold, and cool when it is warm. These fibers include wool, silk, cotton and, if it is combined with other fibers to resist wrinkling, linen. If you are investing in your first suit, choose a lightweight wool, such as a fine gabardine, wool crepe or jersey knit since you'll be able to wear it almost all year round. For warm weather dressing, look for a suit in a heavy silk or a blend of silk/wool, silk/linen or silk/cotton.

The jacket should be well-constructed and have a strongly de-fined shape. Pay attention to the details: The stitching should be even and preferably handsewn; the buttonholes cleanly finished, and the but-tons of a quality material, not cheap and flashy. (Of course, you can always change the buttons after you buy the jacket.) The style of the jacket depends upon your figure and your taste. You may choose a classic blazer, either single- or double-breasted, or one with a shawl collar, cardigan neckline or V-neckline. Whatever style you choose, the sleeves should be long enough to reach your wristbone yet allow your cuffs to show through, and the bottom of the jacket low enough to cover your blouse completely. If you are short, you may want a jacket that stops at your hipbone so that you don't appear to be swallowed up in your clothes. If you are tall, however, you may want one that covers your derrière. No matter what your height, do make sure that the jacket is long enough and doesn't break in the middle of your derrière since this gives a very unflattering look.

Keep in mind that you look most effective in clothes that are attractive on you. No one style is right for everybody, and you ought to have more than one style in your wardrobe. If not, your clothes will become terribly boring. By including a variety of styles in the jackets, skirts, blouses and dresses you buy, you'll feel as if you're wearing a different outfit every day. If you own only blazers or cardigans, or ex-clusively one style of anything, even in different fabrics, you may feel as if you are wearing the same clothes day in and day out.

When buying skirts, look for a variety of styles. For the Corporate profile choose skirts that are slim but not skinny, or full but not flaring. The perfectly straight skirt has an economical look, but don't buy one without looking in a three way mirror. There's something unsightly about a woman in a skinny skirt with her belly sticking out in the front and her derrière sticking out behind. Choose a skirt that has enough fullness so that it fits you well and gives you a long, smooth, clean line. If the style is narrow, look for one with some type of small slit or kick pleat as this allows you to walk gracefully and move easily. Remember that you won't be spending your whole day behind a desk. You have to climb stairs, get in and out of cars, and sit down and stand up, and you'll want to do it all comfortably.

A slightly modified version of the slim skirt is the dirndl shape. This has some shirring or pleating at the waist which gives it more fabric and fullness. The dirndl is usually an easy style to wear and looks flattering on any figure. By all means when you are buying a skirt, look for one that has pockets. They give you a place to put your hands when you are standing about or talking to someone. Men have always had pockets and used them. Pockets are a definite plus in any woman's clothing strategy. One caveat, however: Pockets usually come on more expensive clothes as they cost more for the manufacturer to include.

A third skirt style is one with pleats, preferably hip-stitched, narrow knife pleats, or flat box pleats. These give the clean look of a slim skirt but allow for more facile movement. Pleated skirts generally look best on women who are narrow through the hips as they tend to emphasize that part of the body. They are particularly attractive on thin women who may need some extra fullness.

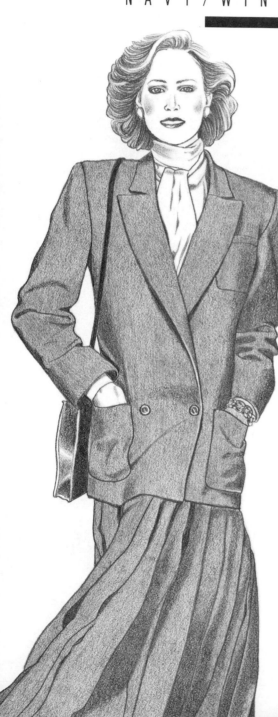

TRADITIONAL CORPORATE CAPSULE: NAVY/WINE

A workable Capsule has at least twelve pieces in it, including skirts, jackets, blouses, dresses (and sometimes pants, although they aren't appropriate in the Corporate profile). This capsule is based on *navy and wine* and has *three jackets, three skirts, four blouses and two dresses*. As you will see, these twelve pieces make more than forty different outfits.

In this traditional Corporate Capsule in navy and wine we chose three different jackets and three different skirts which give three matched suit looks. They might be manufactured by Evan Picone, Saint Laurie or Harvé Benard. The first suit is navy, an excellent color to use for your interviews and a promising introduction to your Capsule. A second suit is wine, and a third is a navy and wine tweed. Remember that in building your Capsule, you should have a diversity of styles. If one jacket is a blazer, another might be a cardigan or a V-neck. If one skirt is slim, look for others that are pleated or dirndl styles. When you're buying these clothes, try them on with the other components so that you are sure they work together. You should be able to combine them in terms of color, fabric and shape.

The navy jacket is in a classic double-breasted blazer style. The matching skirt is pleated. These two pieces are combined to make a very elegant suit which can be used for interviews, conferences, presentations and major meetings. But you can also use them with the other components in the Capsule for maximum versatility. The second jacket is in wine. This time we'll choose a different shape, a cardigan style jacket with navy and wine braided trim. The slim skirt is in the matching wine color. Again, the jacket and skirt are combined to make a smart, serious suit but one without the solemnity of the navy version. The third jacket is a navy and wine tweed. The style of it is a single-breasted, wide lapel jacket in a slightly shorter length. Here again, we'll vary the shapes by using a matching tweed skirt in a dirndl style. This makes another professional and appropriate Corporate suit.

Each of the jackets described above can be combined with any of the skirts. Of course, the navy jacket goes with the navy skirt. It also goes with the wine skirt, and if you are concerned about giving it a pulled together look, you might add a wine-colored scarf, belt or blouse to the outfit. By using any of these wine-colored pieces, you are picking up the color of the skirt and tying it in with the jacket, thereby unifying the look of the ensemble. The navy jacket also works with the tweed skirt. This time, by using a navy belt or blouse, or a navy and wine print scarf, you'll be giving the outfit a coordinated attitude rather than a separates look. In a similar way, the wine jacket goes with the wine skirt, the navy skirt and the tweed skirt. And the tweed jacket works with the tweed skirt, the navy skirt and the wine skirt.

We use four blouses in this Capsule, all with long sleeves, including at least one white blouse. Many women have trouble getting their clothes to look coordinated and often the problem is a lack of white blouses. A white blouse can pull your outfits together and it goes with just about every skirt and jacket. White blouses give you the greatest flexibility and possibility for variety, and the clean simplicity that you want in the Corporate Capsule.

The four blouses include: two white blouses, one in a shirt style with a convertible collar that can be worn open or closed, and a second white blouse with a small pointed collar that comes with a detachable bow; a navy blouse with a collar that can be worn several ways and also has a detachable bow; and a wine blouse with a pleated front, convertible shirt collar style. Each of these blouses can be worn with any of the skirt and jacket combinations. You can see that by varying the blouse, you can dramatically change the look of each outfit.

Two dresses round out the last components of the traditional Corporate Capsule. We chose simple tailored styles that can be worn on their own, with the three different jackets, and even with the blouses underneath. The first style is a navy V-neck straight dress with long sleeves and gold buttons. The second dress is in wine, the same color as the jacket and in a shirtdress style. The most conservative way of

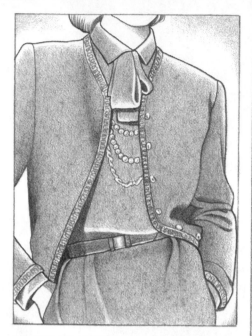

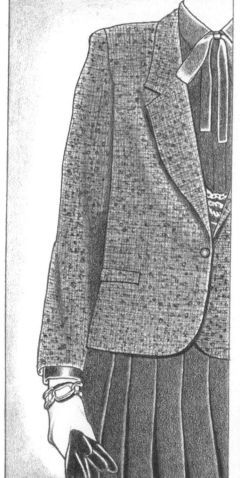

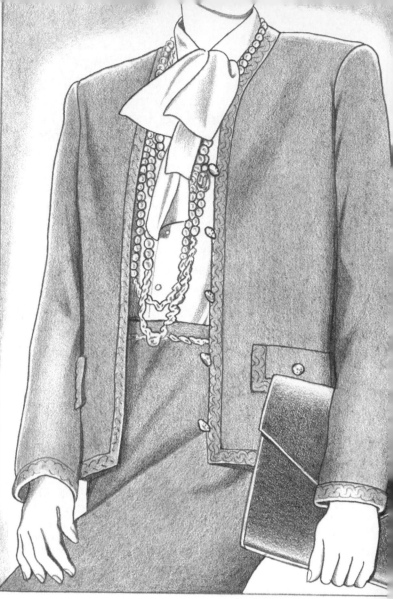

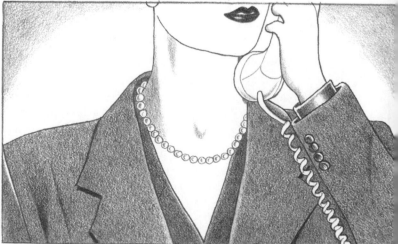

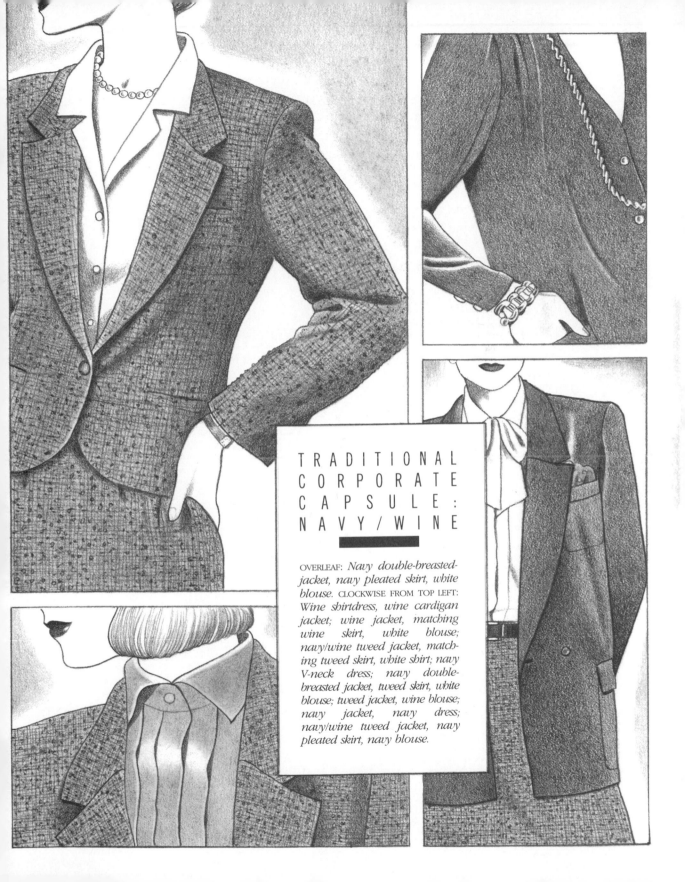

TRADITIONAL CORPORATE CAPSULE: NAVY/WINE

OVERLEAF: *Navy double-breasted-jacket, navy pleated skirt, white blouse.* CLOCKWISE FROM TOP LEFT: *Wine shirtdress, wine cardigan jacket; wine jacket, matching wine skirt, white blouse; navy/wine tweed jacket, matching tweed skirt, white shirt; navy V-neck dress; navy double-breasted jacket, tweed skirt, white blouse; tweed jacket, wine blouse; navy jacket, navy dress; navy/wine tweed jacket, navy pleated skirt, navy blouse.*

wearing both dresses is to coordinate them with the matching jackets. The two dresses are tailored and crisp enough, however, to be appropriate even when worn without a jacket.

These then are the twelve pieces of the Capsule:

- ☐ Navy double-breasted jacket
- ☐ Navy pleated skirt
- ☐ Wine cardigan jacket
- ☐ Wine slim skirt
- ☐ Navy and wine tweed single-breasted jacket
- ☐ Navy and wine tweed dirndl skirt
- ☐ White shirt
- ☐ White bow blouse
- ☐ Navy blouse
- ☐ Wine blouse
- ☐ Navy V-neck dress
- ☐ Wine shirtdress

As you can see on the chart, these pieces are all interrelated and add up to more than two months of different outfits.

A second traditional Corporate Capsule is based on a combination of *navy and gray*. Since many women feel most comfortable wearing suits, this Capsule includes *four jackets, four skirts and four blouses.* There are four matched suits plus enough other coordinated outfits so that these twelve pieces can be combined to make forty-eight different looks.

A very conservative color combination, navy and gray is quite effective for those women who are in extremely traditional, male-oriented organizations. But these two colors need not always look bland. The style of the clothes has as much impact as the colors. In addition, the blouses and accessories that you wear can change the look. There are navy and gray clothes that are made by traditional manufacturers such as Harvé Benard, Stanley Blacker or Evan Picone, but you can also find these colors in the collections of Christian Dior or even Yves Saint Laurent.

The first outfit in this Capsule is a navy suit. We'll choose a classic style single-breasted jacket with a shawl collar. The matching navy skirt is a slim style with a kick pleat. This matched suit is excellent for interviews, conferences, presentations and important meetings.

A second matched suit in gray is equally effective for high-powered occasions. This suit has a longer V-neck cardigan jacket and a matching pleated skirt. Now you have two different styles of jackets and two different styles of skirts; both of these suits project a high-powered aura.

Both the navy jacket and the gray jacket can be worn with the navy skirt and

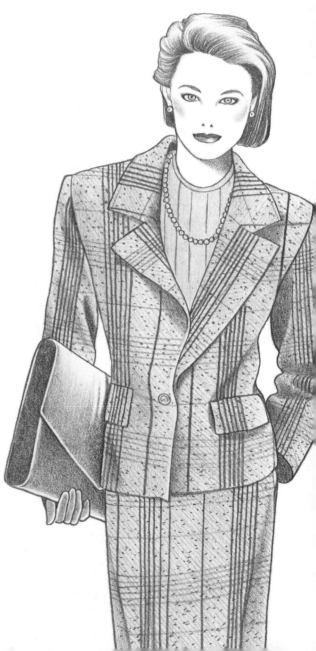

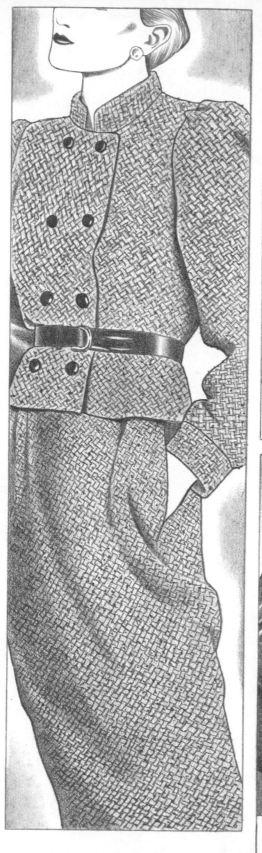
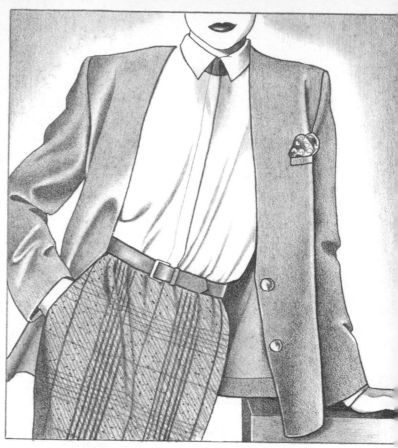
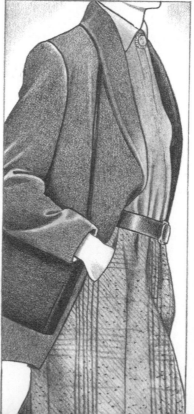
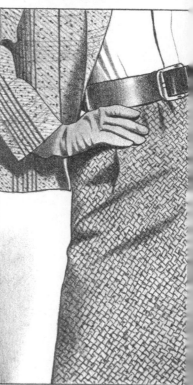

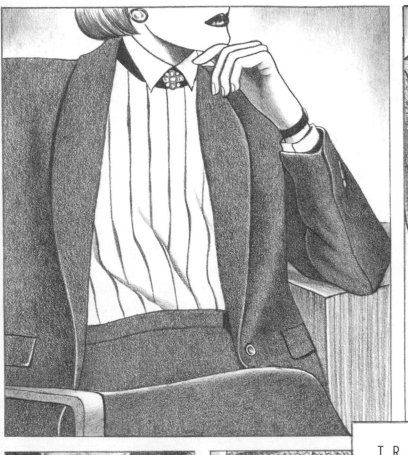

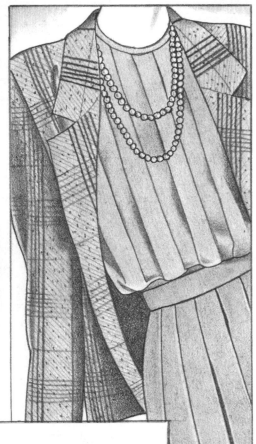

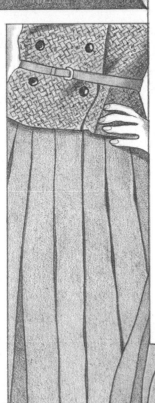

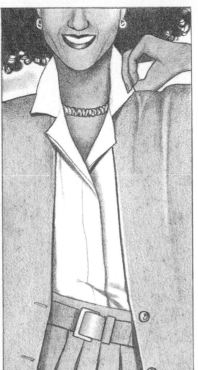

TRADITIONAL CORPORATE CAPSULE: NAVY/GRAY

OVERLEAF: *Navy/gray/white menswear plaid jacket, matching plaid skirt, gray blouse.* CLOCKWISE FROM LEFT: *Navy/gray tweed jacket, matching tweed skirt; gray V-neck jacket, plaid skirt, white blouse; navy shawl collar jacket, matching navy skirt, yellow blouse; plaid jacket, gray pleated skirt, gray blouse; tweed jacket, gray pleated skirt; gray V-neck jacket, gray skirt, white blouse; plaid jacket, navy/gray tweed skirt, white blouse; navy jacket, plaid skirt, curry blouse.*

the gray skirt. To pull the look together, use a scarf, belt or blouse. For example, take the navy jacket and gray pleated skirt and show a small gray scarf in the blazer pocket. A gray blouse gives a finished look. If you put the gray jacket with the navy skirt, you can wear a navy scarf at the neck or wrap the jacket with a navy belt and either of these accessories work to coordinate the outfit.

The third jacket is a navy and gray tweed in a double-breasted style. The matching skirt is made of the same navy and gray tweed and cut in a slim style. Of course, together these make an attractive, authoritative suit. They also work well with the other components in the Capsule. The tweed jacket goes with the navy skirt as well as the gray skirt, and the tweed skirt can be combined with the navy or gray jacket.

The fourth jacket in this Capsule is a navy, gray and white menswear plaid in a single-breasted style. The matching navy, gray and white plaid skirt is a slim dirndl. This gives you a fourth serious suit appropriate for meetings and conferences. Just as with the other styles, these components can be interchanged with the rest of the Capsule. The plaid jacket works with its own skirt, the navy skirt, the gray skirt and the tweed skirt. Likewise, the plaid skirt can be worn with its matching jacket, the navy jacket, the gray jacket and the tweed jacket. Don't be concerned about mixing tweeds and plaids; keep in mind that if the shades of the colors are the same, they'll not only work together, but will lend an interesting, sophisticated look.

There are four long-sleeve blouses to go with the jackets and skirts. The first blouse is in white, and has a convertible shirt collar. It will give any of the outfits a crisp and efficient look. To add a little interest to the outfits we'll also use other colors in the blouses. The second blouse is a pleated front shirt style in yellow. Another is in a curry shade with a versatile collar and the fourth, a jewel neck in gray, gives a soft look. Each of the blouses can be used with any of the outfits.

The navy and gray Corporate Capsule consists of these twelve pieces:

- ☐ Navy single-breasted jacket with shawl collar
- ☐ Navy slim skirt
- ☐ Gray V-neck jacket
- ☐ Gray pleated skirt
- ☐ Navy and gray tweed double-breasted jacket
- ☐ Navy and gray tweed slim skirt

☐ Navy, gray and white plaid single-breasted jacket
☐ Navy, gray and white plaid dirndl skirt
☐ White blouse
☐ Gray blouse
☐ Curry blouse
☐ Yellow blouse

This well-suited wardrobe will also take you through two working months with a different outfit every day.

This Capsule can also be combined with the navy and wine Capsule because the colors are compatible. This will give you many more looks as you work the gray and wine components together. Later on, if you decide to add a brighter accent to your wardrobe, you might introduce more of the curry or the yellow color. These colors work well with the navy, the gray, and the wine and bring another dimension altogether to your dressing.

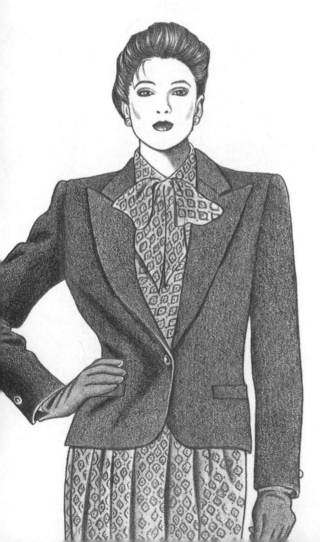

The third Corporate Capsule is based around black and beige. It can be adapted to all-weather dressing because of its dark and light looks, and therefore is perfect for businesswomen who travel frequently. Of course, the kinds of fabrics you choose are important. Consider lightweight wools and heavy silks along with blends of silk, wool and linen if you want clothes that can be worn from winter through summer.

This contemporary *black and beige Capsule* has *three jackets, four skirts, four blouses and one dress*. It includes three matched suits along with two dress looks, all of which are appropriate for the Corporate profile. Clothes from Liz Claiborne, Spitalnick and Anne Klein II usually fit the contemporary image.

The first jacket is in black and has a one button closing with peaked lapels. Its matching black skirt is slim but with some softness under the waistband. Together these components make a crisp, efficient Corporate suit that has power and authority with feminine styling.

The second jacket is in beige. It is in a double-breasted style. This jacket combines well with a matching beige skirt in a box pleated style and makes another effective Corporate suit. The four pieces can also be interchanged so that the black jacket is worn with the beige skirt and the beige jacket is worn with the black skirt. Just as we did with the other Capsules, we can bring a coordinated look to these pieces by adding a scarf, a belt or a blouse.

The third jacket is in a subtle black and beige check. This is a single-breasted blazer style. It makes an authoritative and attractive suit when combined with its matching black and beige checked slim wrap skirt. Naturally, this checked jacket can be worn with the two solid color skirts, the black and the beige. The checked skirt too can be coordinated with either the black jacket or the beige jacket.

To give some variety to this Capsule add a black and beige paisley skirt in a pleated style. This skirt can be combined with a matching black and beige paisley blouse that has a detachable bow. When worn together, they give the look of an elegant, tailored dress. Put any of the jackets with it—either the black, the beige or the plaid—and the outfit is authoritative and serious enough to look appropriate in the corporate world. In addition to acting as a dress, these paisley components can work with the rest of the Capsule for other looks.

There are three other blouses in this Capsule: a white blouse in a convertible collar style; a beige blouse with a stock tie; and a cinnamon color blouse with a detachable bow. All of these blouses work with any of the skirt and jacket combinations we discussed.

The last piece is the dress, a black V-neck sleeveless style. It can be worn as a jumper using any of the blouses underneath. The dress goes with any of the jackets so that it can be worn to meetings and other similar occasions. It can also be worn without a jacket and still look appropriate, or spruced up to make for perfect evening attire.

The twelve pieces in this black and beige Corporate Capsule give you fifty different outfits. The components are:

- [ ] Black one button jacket
- [ ] Black slim skirt
- [ ] Beige double-breasted jacket
- [ ] Beige pleated skirt
- [ ] Black and beige checked jacket
- [ ] Black and beige checked skirt
- [ ] Black and beige paisley skirt
- [ ] Black and beige paisley blouse
- [ ] White blouse
- [ ] Beige blouse
- [ ] Cinnamon blouse
- [ ] Black V-neck dress

This is another Capsule that takes you through two working months with a different look every day.

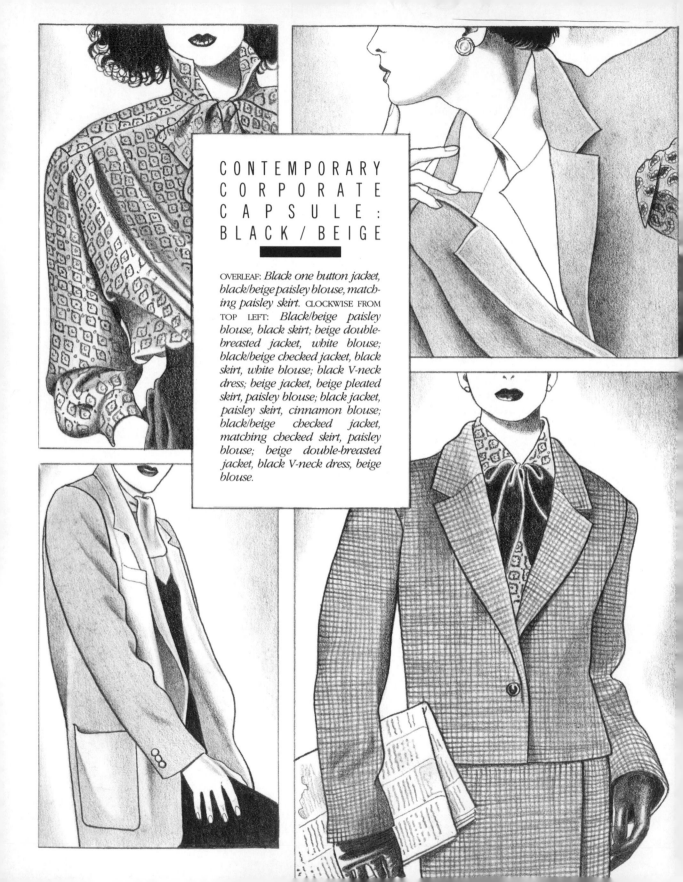

CONTEMPORARY CORPORATE CAPSULE: BLACK / BEIGE

OVERLEAF: *Black one button jacket, black/beige paisley blouse, matching paisley skirt.* CLOCKWISE FROM TOP LEFT: *Black/beige paisley blouse, black skirt; beige double-breasted jacket, white blouse; black/beige checked jacket, black skirt, white blouse; black V-neck dress; beige jacket, beige pleated skirt, paisley blouse; black jacket, paisley skirt, cinnamon blouse; black/beige checked jacket, matching checked skirt, paisley blouse; beige double-breasted jacket, black V-neck dress, beige blouse.*

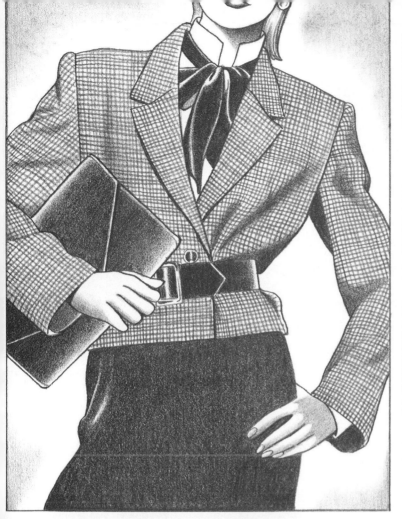

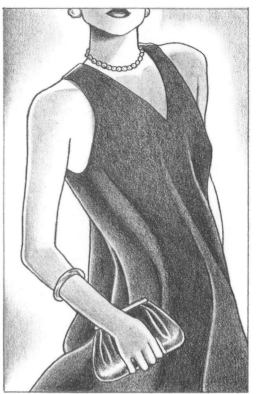

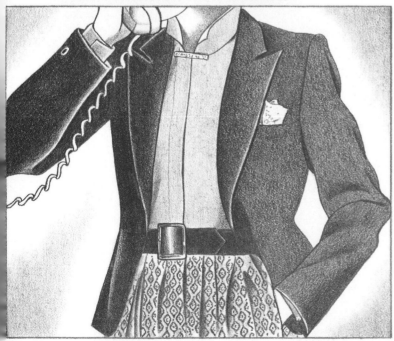

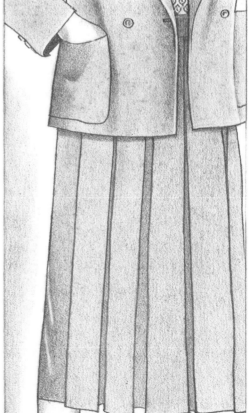

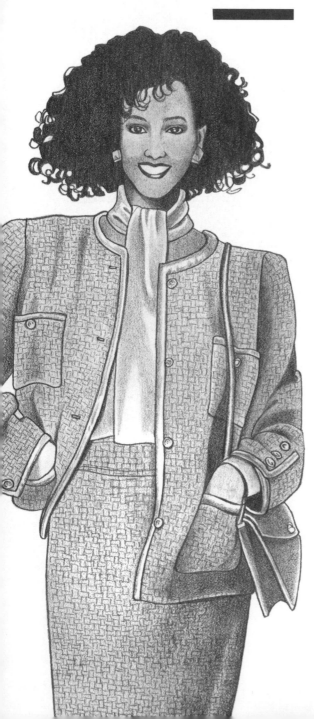

The fourth Corporate Capsule combines *gray and brown* in both suit and dress styles. There are *two matched suits, three dresses, one with its own jacket, and four blouses.*

The first jacket is a gray cardigan edged with brown trim. The matching gray skirt is slim with kick pleats. This suit makes a very attractive, appropriate interview suit that is classic without being boring. You can find this look from Castleberry, St. John, Adolfo and Chanel.

The second jacket is in a brown and gray subtle plaid. It is a double-breasted blazer. Its matching brown and gray plaid skirt has hip-stitched pleats. This gives you another serious suit with a bit more fabric interest than the solid color ones. The plaid jacket also goes with the gray skirt and the gray jacket goes with the plaid skirt.

The first dress in this Capsule is in gray in a shirtdress style. This classic, tailored look is worn with either the gray jacket or the plaid jacket for an authoritative, assertive look. It is also worn without the jacket and still looks serious and businesslike.

The second dress is solid brown, sleeveless, with a jewel neck. It comes with its own matching brown one button blazer jacket that goes with the other pieces in the Capsule. This dress too can be worn with or without the jacket, or with any of the other jackets. Because it is sleeveless it also looks attractive with any of the blouses worn underneath.

The third dress is a jewel neckline button-front style in a subtle brown and gray stripe. It too can be worn with any of the jackets or on its own. Because of the jewel neckline, it too can be worn with any of the blouses underneath.

The four long-sleeve blouses include white and colors. The first blouse, in white, is a pleated front shirt style. The second blouse is a brick color with a detachable bow. The third blouse is in gray in a stock tie style. The fourth blouse is in yellow with a convertible collar. These blouses work with all of the skirt and jacket or dress combinations.

This gray and brown Capsule includes:

- [ ] Gray cardigan jacket
- [ ] Gray slim skirt
- [ ] Gray and brown plaid jacket
- [ ] Gray and brown plaid skirt
- [ ] Gray shirtdress
- [ ] Brown jewel neck dress
- [ ] Brown blazer jacket
- [ ] Gray and brown striped dress
- [ ] White blouse
- [ ] Brick blouse
- [ ] Gray blouse
- [ ] Yellow blouse

These twelve pieces make forty different outfits for a different look every day of two working months.

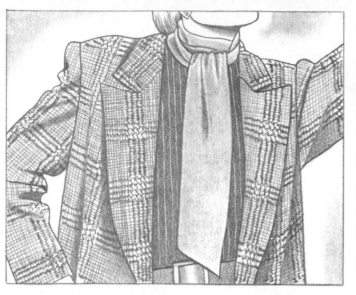

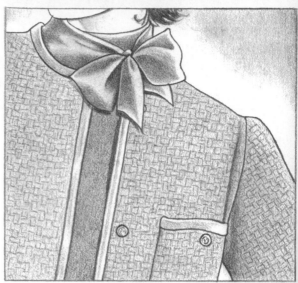

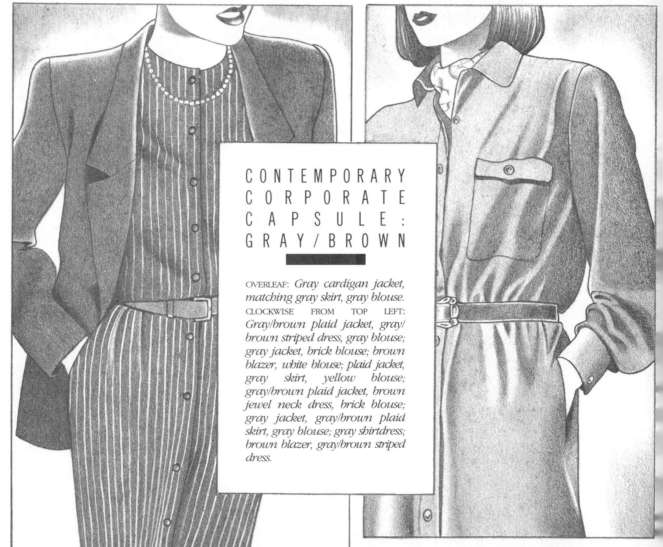

CONTEMPORARY CORPORATE CAPSULE: GRAY/BROWN

OVERLEAF: *Gray cardigan jacket, matching gray skirt, gray blouse.*
CLOCKWISE FROM TOP LEFT: *Gray/brown plaid jacket, gray/ brown striped dress, gray blouse; gray jacket, brick blouse; brown blazer, white blouse; plaid jacket, gray skirt, yellow blouse; gray/brown plaid jacket, brown jewel neck dress, brick blouse; gray jacket, gray/brown plaid skirt, gray blouse; gray shirtdress; brown blazer, gray/brown striped dress.*

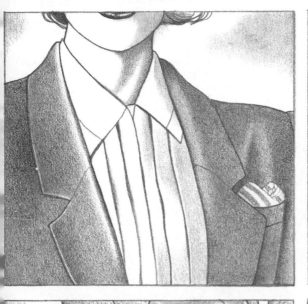

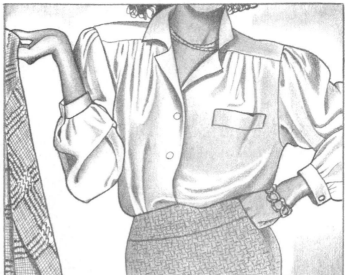

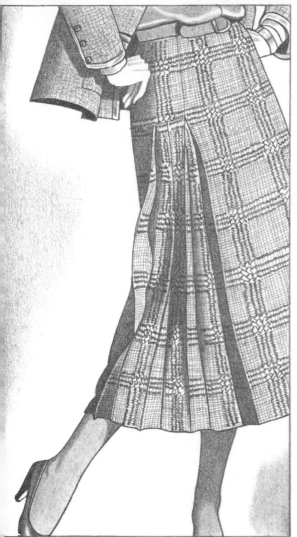

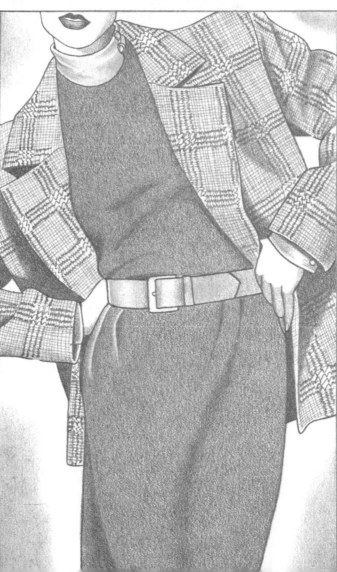

ACCESSORIES FOR THE CORPORATE CAPSULE

Because any clothing Capsule is based on two colors, it allows you to work with a minimum number of shoes, handbags, belts, scarves and jewelry. Since the leather goods and the jewelry can be expensive items, it is reassuring to know that your long term purchases in these categories can be kept to a small number. These basic accessories work with all of the components in your Capsule. Since you don't need many individual pieces, buy the best you can afford. You'll find that these investments, once again, give you the best return on your money and time spent. They help you get high productivity from your wardrobe and an appearance that expresses your appreciation of quality work and attention to detail.

A Capsule of accessories should include about twelve basic pieces:
- ☐ Two pairs of shoes
- ☐ One handbag
- ☐ Two belts
- ☐ Two pairs of earrings
- ☐ Two necklaces
- ☐ Three scarves

These are the pieces you know you can count on to pull together any outfit in your Capsule. When you're rushing to get dressed, you'll be able to accessorize any outfit quickly and with the confidence that what you wear speaks well for you. A Capsule of accessories can save you the agony of what shoes to wear with what dress, the inconvenience of changing handbags and losing keys, and the difficulty of deciding on earrings, necklaces or scarves. Once you have acquired these basic pieces, you may choose to supplement your accessories Capsule. Then you'll have the chance to bring in other colors, amusing jewelry or interesting belts. But be sure to begin with the best basic pieces you can buy. You'll find they can last a lifetime.

The accessories in the Corporate Capsule reflect the same attributes as your clothing: precise, high quality pieces that have a minimum of fussiness or detail. They have simple, clean lines, and are made of the best materials. You may not be as fastidious or extravagant as fashion expert Diana Vreeland, who polishes the soles of her shoes, but bear in mind that your accessories do speak for you.

One of the most expensive accessory items is shoes. The cost of a good pair of shoes is about as much as any good clothing item, so the investment should be as careful and considered. For a Corporate profile, the best shoes are simple pumps or slingbacks with closed toes. In hot weather, you may decide on modified versions of these shoes, such as a style with small open toes. The best heel height is about two inches. Avoid bare sandals, open backs, casual styles, or any shoes that make noise when you walk in them. Since a pump style can include anything in a closed shoe from British walking brogues to elegantly simple high-heeled shoes, there is plenty of room for variety in your footwear. Try on different styles with your outfits to see how they change the mood of your clothes.

Two pairs of shoes are all you need as a base for your Capsule. One reason many women overload on their shoe purchases is that they aren't sure what colors go with what clothes. By working with two Capsule colors, you can avoid all those unnecessary shoes in your closet. You'll also find that when you travel, you won't need so many shoes; you can easily get by almost anywhere with one pair of walking shoes and one pair of dressier pumps. This saves space in your suitcase and cuts down on the weight of your bag which can be a blessing. In this chapter on Corporate Capsules, I outlined four color combinations. The first is navy and wine. A pair of shoes in navy and another pair in wine work with all of those outfits. The second Capsule is based on navy and gray. Here too the neutral colors can be interchanged, so that one pair of shoes in navy and one pair in gray work with all of your clothes. In the black and beige Capsule, a pair of shoes in black and a pair in beige is perfect. Consider choosing the first pair in black, and the second in a beige and black combination. This classic, elegant shoe has never gone out of style and always looks smart. Sometimes available in other color combinations such as navy and wine, it might be a good alternative for that Capsule as well. The fourth Corporate Capsule is based on gray and brown, and a pair of simple pumps or closed-toe slingbacks in each of these colors works well.

When you're buying shoes, look for good quality leather, suede or skin. They look better, retain their shape and their color, and last longer than cheap imitations. Because you're buying classic styles, you may be able to take advantage of sales on some famous-maker shoes such as Ferragamo or Magli, which are usually held twice a year. I know many women who wait for those sales and stock up on their favorite classic styles. There are other good quality manufacturers who are not quite as expensive. Anne Klein, Evan Picone and Delman all make well-styled, classic shoes.

The handbag of a Corporate woman says a great deal about her. It is something that people see almost immediately and usually take note of, and it is worn regularly. Look for a classic style in the best leather you can afford, and choose a bag that is not too large. If you carry a briefcase, attaché or portfolio, then select a handbag that fits inside. This is one of the best ways to keep a sleek, precise appearance from turning into a sloppy one. If your male colleagues carry nothing at all or simply attachés, it adversely affects your power image to be seen as a person who must carry many bags. When going out to lunch or dinner, remove your handbag and leave your case at the office. Your briefcase is also perfect to carry extra accessories to the office if you are going out at night. Some attachés and portfolios even come with a small matching handbag inside. The neatest shapes to look for are envelope styles, clutch bags or small shoulder bags which sometimes come with detachable straps. Coach, Anne Klein and Susan Gail all make attractive handbags in these styles. At a higher price point, Chanel, Fendi and Bottega Veneta are excellent options.

One handbag is all you need to work with your Capsule. Choose one of the colors from your clothes Capsule; it can be navy or wine, black or gray, beige or black, gray or brown. If you go out a great deal after work, pick the darker color in your Capsule as dark colors generally have a dressier look than lighter shades. You may argue that a smaller bag won't hold all of the cosmetics and assorted items that you tend to carry. It may be time to clean out your bag and keep some of these things in a separate drawer of your desk. If you do, put them in a neat cosmetic case so that if someone accidentally opens your drawer they won't discover a scaled-down version of a variety store.

The accessories Capsule includes two belts, one in each color of your clothes Capsule. Once again, look for high quality leathers, suedes or skins in simple styles. The most classic belts are about one and a half inches wide with a self or brass buckle. Wearing a belt gives a finished look to an outfit, so be sure to include these in your Capsule.

Look for natural fibers when you choose your scarves. Good quality silk scarves serve you for years and years. Many women find that the scarves they own are impractical or impossible to tie, such as small squares which are not adaptable to many ways of tieing. Instead, choose scarves that are oblongs. I have found these to be the most flexible. You can use an oblong shape to make a bow or a muffler, or to even wrap your waist. At least one and preferably two of your scarves should be in a Capsule color. A scarf is literally one of the best ways to tie an outfit together. It also makes a good accent, brightening an outfit or adding some drama to it, so look for another scarf in a completely different color from your Capsule combination. For example, with the navy and wine group, think about mustard or pink or teal. With the navy and gray, you may choose an accent of red or yellow or hot pink. With the black and beige, think about toast or rust or even red. With the gray and brown, an accent color in purple or teal or orange works well.

Your jewelry should be as simple as the other pieces in your accessories Capsule. Nevertheless, you can make an elegant statement about yourself with the right jewelry. You can show flair without being flamboyant. If you wear earrings, look for styles that rest on your ears. Don't buy anything that dangles or moves; it can be terribly distracting and take attention away from what you are saying. Choose two simple styles, one in pearl, the other in gold or silver, which work with all of your outfits. The pearl has the dressiest look, the silver the most casual, although all three are appropriate for work.

If you are including two necklaces in this group, look for the same materials as your earrings. Since this is the base of your accessories Capsule, you'll find it gives you a coordinated, precise look. Pearls and gold are the most practical combination as they can be worn separately or together. A strand of pearls that can be doubled is the most useful length to buy. In all of your accessories, simplicity and elegance are the key elements that give you a feminine, professional look.

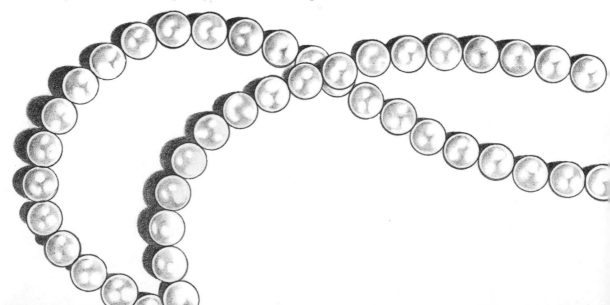

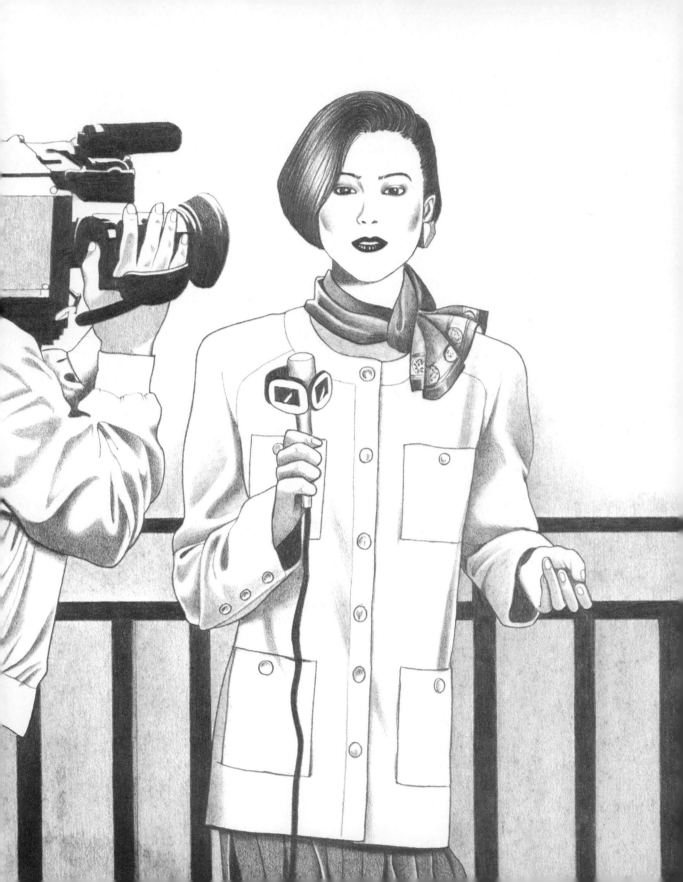

CHAPTER VII

The Communicator Capsule

The Communicator has the freedom to dress with lots of variety and verve. Her clothes can range from serious to amusing, from structured to relaxed, from solid and dark to patterned and bright. Her appearance is an amalgam of her personality, her organization's image, her position and her audience's language. Because there is much more diversity between these elements than there is within the Corporate profile, the Communicator has much more latitude in the ways she may express herself. That's not to say that the Corporate woman isn't dressing to suit her own personality; she should be. The matched

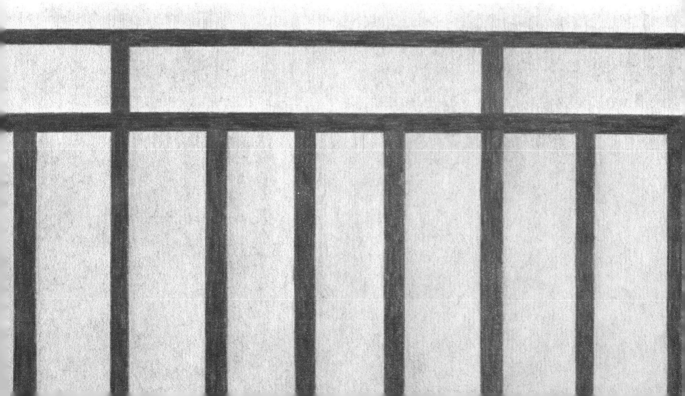

suit or tailored clothes of the Corporate Capsule can be as comfortable for the Corporate personality as the less constructed and less constricting clothes are for the Communicator.

PUBLIC SPEAKING AND TELEVISION APPEARANCES

All women should be familiar with the clothing cues of the Communicator. Corporate and Creative women too are frequently asked to speak in public or appear on television and, on these occasions, should know how to put together a Communicator Capsule appropriate for their audience and their message.

If you have been asked to speak, then you are probably considered an authority on a subject matter. An audience usually willingly vests authority in a speaker: They want you to be an authority and to assert yourself. If you have listened to speeches, then you know there is nothing worse than a wishy-washy speaker who isn't sure of her subject matter or herself. By all means, look like the authority you are. Look assertive, but not intimidating. Your clothes should express that attitude.

Good speakers often begin with an amusing story or an anecdote, and you can do the same with your clothing. If your suit is a dark color, choose a bright-colored blouse or striking scarf or necklace to lighten up your outfit. This also adds a feeling of friendliness on your part. If your suit is in a bright color, you'll immediately stand out, express confidence in yourself and indicate affability with your audience.

For anyone appearing on television or in front of a large audience, it is essential that your clothing feels comfortable and that you are completely familiar with it. As an account executive, you might wear a new outfit on the day of a major meeting. In fact, it will make you feel terrific to appear at a presentation in new clothes. But if you're appearing on television, beware. Be totally familiar with the clothes you wear; this is not the time for surprises. Know how the jacket feels and looks when it's buttoned as well as unbuttoned. Know where the hem of the skirt hits your leg when you're sitting and standing. Know how the collar of your blouse falls on your jacket, where your skirt pockets are when standing, and how your whole outfit looks from the front, the side and the back.

Color is a big factor in how you look on camera. Clear bright colors such as blues and reds, and even ivory, are excellent. Dark colors

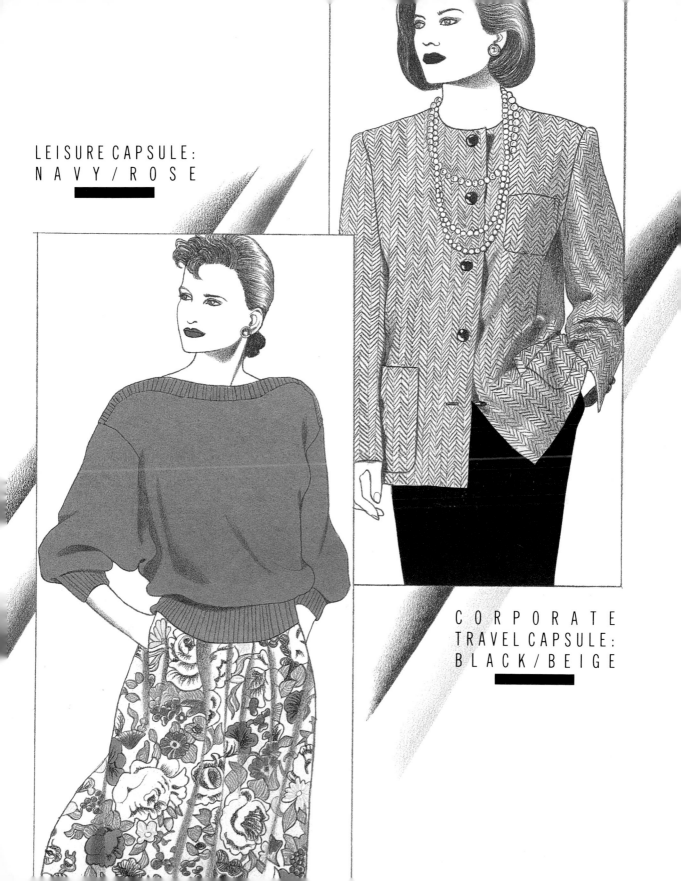

LEISURE CAPSULE:
N A V Y / R O S E

C O R P O R A T E
TRAVEL CAPSULE:
B L A C K / B E I G E

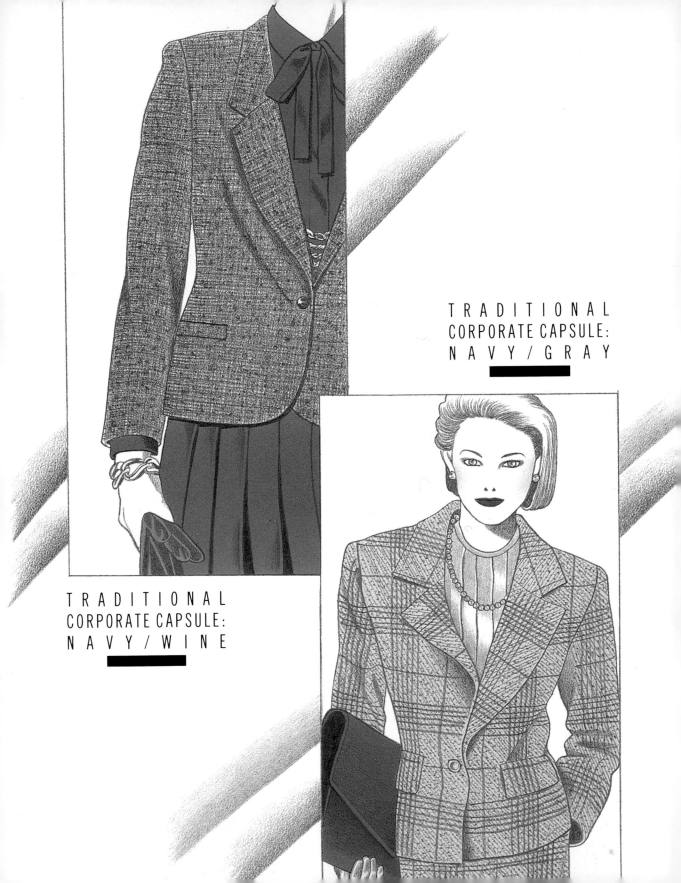

TRADITIONAL
CORPORATE CAPSULE:
N A V Y / G R A Y

TRADITIONAL
CORPORATE CAPSULE:
N A V Y / W I N E

CONTEMPORARY
CORPORATE CAPSULE:
BLACK / BEIGE

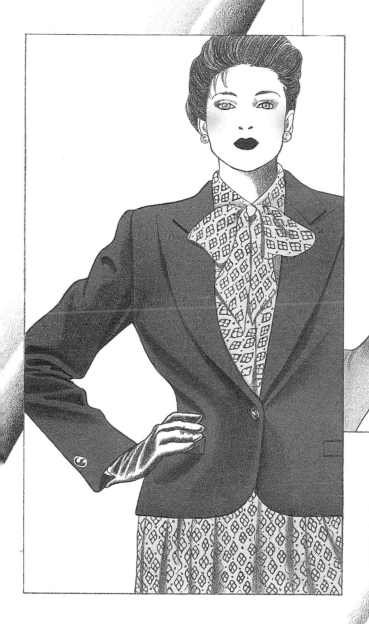

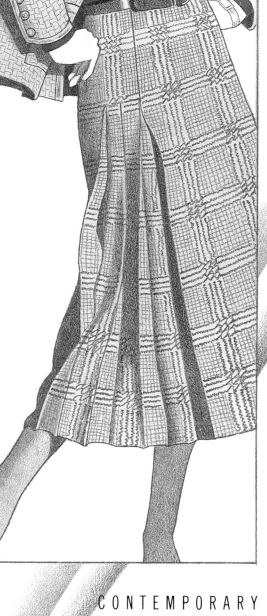

CONTEMPORARY
CORPORATE CAPSULE:
GRAY / BROWN

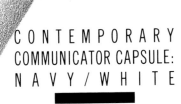

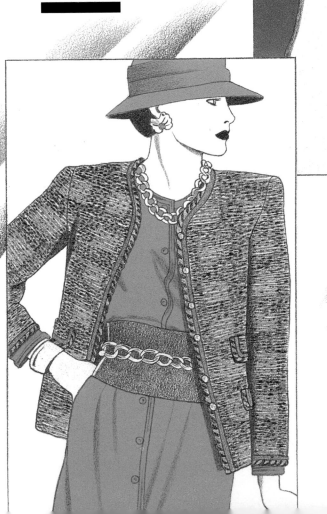

TRADITIONAL
COMMUNICATOR CAPSULE:
WINE / GREEN

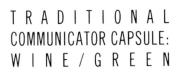

CONTEMPORARY
COMMUNICATOR CAPSULE:
NAVY / WHITE

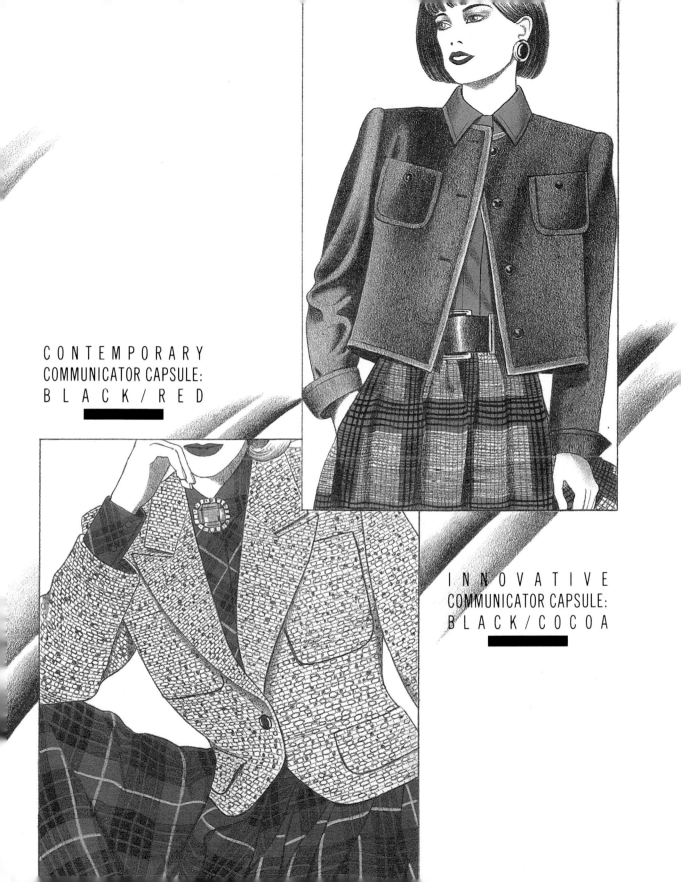

CONTEMPORARY
COMMUNICATOR CAPSULE:
B L A C K / R E D

I N N O V A T I V E
COMMUNICATOR CAPSULE:
B L A C K / C O C O A

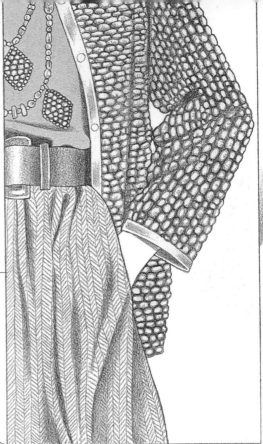

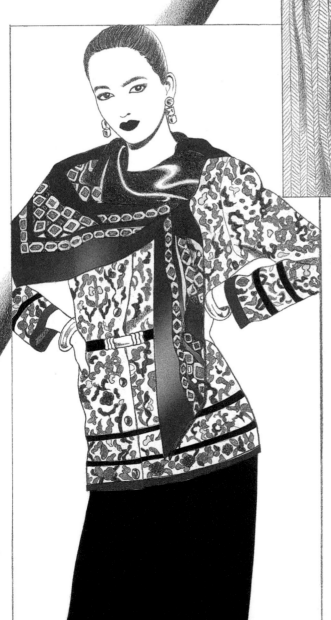

I N N O V A T I V E
CREATIVE CAPSULE:
C A M E L / C R E A M

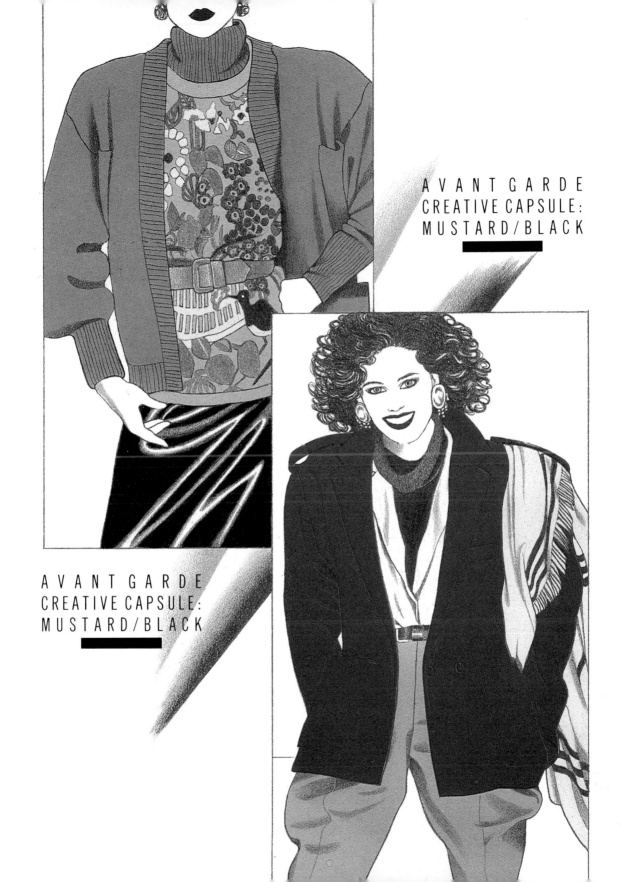

AVANT GARDE
CREATIVE CAPSULE:
MUSTARD/BLACK

AVANT GARDE
CREATIVE CAPSULE:
MUSTARD/BLACK

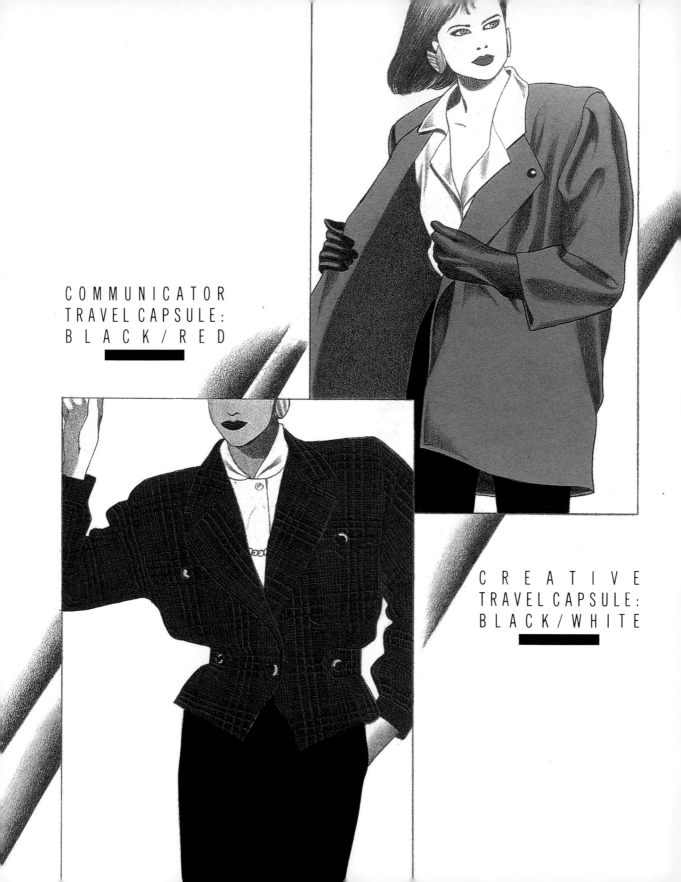

COMMUNICATOR
TRAVEL CAPSULE:
BLACK / RED

CREATIVE
TRAVEL CAPSULE:
BLACK / WHITE

such as navy and gray work well, especially if there's some contrast in an accessory. However, black clothes don't show up clearly. Murky colors tend to make you look murky too, and pastels wash away. Solid colors look sharp and clear, whereas prints or patterns can look confusing if they are large, too jumpy if they are small.

The most effective clothes for the camera are simple styles with clean lines in strong, solid colors. Details on clothes become distracting. Avoid ruffles or bows. Try to dress in a way that relates to your subject matter and your audience. If you're talking about fashion, then by all means, dress the part. Otherwise, stay away from high-fashion styles as they may seem inappropriate. If you're discussing serious issues, dress in a way that gives you authority without being intimidating. For example, if your subject matter is finance, legislation or career planning, then tailored clothes are appropriate. But if you're talking about raising children, growing plants or cooking, then a softer look is probably expected.

Accessories become exaggerated on camera. The most effective jewelry is simple pieces like plain gold earrings and pearls. Anything that makes noise or moves, such as a bracelet or necklace that may hit against your microphone, can be very distracting.

Try on your clothes well in advance of your speech or television appearance. Look for fabrics that are crisp or soft without being clingy or noisy. Wools, silks and cottons usually work well. Some fabrics, such as satin, can rustle and be disturbing. Clingy fabrics such as nylon should also be avoided.

When your clothes look and feel comfortable and attractive, you send your audience a message that you're at ease with yourself, that you're confident and credible. Because you paid attention to your clothes, your audience will pay attention to your words. If, however, you fidget with your clothes, or look awkward in them, your audience will be watching you instead of listening to you. The more positive the impression you make, the more impact your words will have.

The key phrases for the Communicator are competence combined with softness, firmness with friendliness. In the vocabulary of a wardrobe, there are a number of different ways to send these signals. As a Communicator, you may want to alter the emphasis of those signals as your listeners change. The Communicator often has more than one audience. Be aware of who your audience is, and what their expectations are. You may find yourself in front of a housewife one day and a group of professional men and women the next. When in doubt, or if your agenda includes different audiences in the same day, dress to the most professional level. It is far better to be accused of dressing too seriously than of looking amateurish.

FRIENDLY DRESSING

Frequently a Communicator will have professional meetings with people from the corporate world. Therefore, have at least one suit in your wardrobe, a minimum for almost every career woman. You may use that type of structured outfit as often as every day for conferences and meetings, or you may need it as infrequently as once or twice a month for consultations with bankers or business associates. That suit, however, doesn't have to be as constructed or matched as the suit of your Corporate colleagues. You may opt for a dark tone like navy, or choose one in a bright color like raspberry, a menswear pattern or tartan plaid. Similarly, the silhouette may not be as tailored as the Corporate look; select an unconstructed jacket or a softer skirt.

The suit jacket helps give your outfit its authority. If it's in the same fabric as the skirt, it has the most serious look. When the jacket is in a different material, it still looks appropriate and professional if coordinated with the skirt. There are many times when you'll want to take off your jacket, or go without one, so that you look more approachable and friendly. Your blouse then becomes very important. A white blouse signals that you're crisp and efficient while a bright-colored blouse suggests sociability. By not wearing a jacket, you're showing yourself to be open and relaxed. If your audience is dressed casually, this will put you closer to them. They'll feel that you're on their level rather than above them, and they'll find it easier to communicate with you.

A sweater can also have the authoritative effect of a jacket when it is shaped at the shoulders through padding or molding, and when it is made in a thick knit. A sweater looks more relaxed than a jacket, however, and is often the perfect accompaniment to a Communicator's Capsule. When CBS decided to put their evening news anchorman, Dan Rather, in a sweater, it was a deliberate attempt to make him look more relaxed. It was a way of letting the audience identify with him, and it gave him a friendlier, more affable appearance.

Knits can be used in the same way as sweaters. They have the same kind of softness in styling and fabric, and when they're worn in coordinated outfits they can have the finished look of a suit or a dress and jacket. Blouses worn by the Communicator can be more colorful, more textured, and more toned with prints and patterns. Dresses may be menswear tailored or in more relaxed knit styles.

There is plenty of room for color in the Communicator Capsule. You're not limited to neutrals and darks and can take advantage of a broad range of colors, including shades such as hot pinks and brilliant reds, soft pastels, or even quiet tones of beige. You can use colors that contrast and colors that blend. You can keep to solids, or pepper your Capsule with prints, or even combine patterns for a different effect.

This chapter includes four different Communicator Capsules. Each Capsule is based on two colors and includes twelve pieces of clothing. Those components are interrelated so that they all work together. You'll see how to take this small group of clothes and develop a large working wardrobe. The Capsules in this chapter are each decidedly different from the others. You can substitute other color combinations or even other styles in any of the Capsules to give it your individual look. Keep in mind that these Capsules are a good guideline to begin building your Communicator wardrobe.

A TOUCH OF FASHION

As you look at the Capsules in this chapter, think about the clothes that you have and how you might use them. Sometimes we get in a rut with our clothes and don't think about new ways of recycling or updating them. Try new color combinations. See how last year's skirt might work with this year's jacket or a new blouse. By adding one new piece in a more fashionable shape or shade, you can add years of life to your clothes. For example, after several seasons of blacks and grays, I found a bright yellow jacket on sale. It was a little more expensive than my budget warranted, but I decided to make it my one major purchase for the season. The investment paid off. I've worn that jacket with all of the old blacks and grays and suddenly they all look new. You can do the same thing with whatever the latest fashion trend may be. One purchase, like a pale pink blouse, a glittery scarf, an oversized vest or a new pair of bold metal earrings can update last year's look.

There is more room in the Communicator Capsule for fashion

looks. Although advanced fashion designs may be inappropriate for many Communicators, certainly some adaptations are fine. Subtle things, such as the way scarves are worn this year, the size of earrings, the shades of stockings, or the proportions of skirts, jackets and heel heights, all make a difference. As you work with your clothes, look at fashion magazines for ideas. One well-dressed woman I know keeps a bulletin board near her closet. On it she pins up sketches and photographs from *Vogue, W* and other fashion periodicals. That way when she is getting dressed, she has a picture in front of her of what looks new and what looks stylish. That doesn't mean you must slavishly follow this year's fads, but it does help give you a new outlook on your older clothes. It helps you to be more inventive.

By all means, what you wear should look right for you. There is nothing chic or elegant about wearing clothes that don't suit you. It's better to stay with classic shapes that are safe than outrageous styles that make you sorry. *Women's Wear Daily,* the trade newspaper for the fashion industry, calls people who follow fashion trends without thinking about how the clothes look on them "Fashion Victims," and victims they are. Clothing is too big an investment for major mistakes. But do experiment with accessories and with colors. Classic clothing can look boring or it can be beautiful depending upon how you put the pieces together.

The four different Communicator Capsules described here range from traditional to innovative. These Capsules use different color combinations from subtle to strong and include several types of silhouettes from structured suits to sweater knits.

Knits make a strong fashion statement and with good reason: they can look elegant, feel comfortable and pack easily. When fashion designers like Yves Saint Laurent show double knits in their collections, and when American manufacturers like Evan Picone include knits in their sportswear groups, then you know that the fashion picture is moving away from structured clothes into a softer mood. For the Communicator woman who travels, knits are ideal. Keep in mind, however, that they should never cling. Look for knit clothes that have some shape. Double knits do hang better on the body and are not as figure-revealing as slinky, single knits. Although some women do have the figure to carry off a fine knit, most of us look best in styles that fall away from the body or that slide over and cover our lumps and bumps rather than cling to them.

The first Capsule in the Communicator profile combines sophisticated, refined dressing with a color combination of *wine and green*. The pieces include *two jackets, four skirts, one dress, four blouses and one sweater*.

This Capsule is based on the looks of Chanel and Adolfo—suits that have texture and trim, and skirts and blouses that have a refined elegance to them. The first jacket is a tweedy wine knit in a cardigan style that is edged with wine, green and gold braiding. The matching wine tweed skirt is a slim style with kick pleats. This type of suit look is appropriate for business meetings as well as for more formal evening events such as receptions or dinners.

The second jacket is in a plaid that combines the same wine and green shades with a touch of the gold accent. This jacket is in a V-neck cardigan style, longer and fuller than the classic shape of the wine tweed jacket. Use a skirt, in a matching wine and green plaid, that is in a full A-line style. Again, this makes a suit look that is effective for nine-to-five, and on. In addition, the wine jacket can be used with the wine and green plaid skirt, and the wine and green plaid jacket can be worn with the wine skirt.

This Capsule has several dress looks. The first is a skirt and blouse combination in a floral pattern that picks up the Capsule colors of wine and green. The long-sleeve blouse is in a bow neck style. The matching skirt has flat pleats all around. This is a dress look that works from breakfast meetings to dinner and can be accompanied by either the wine tweed or the green and wine plaid jacket. The floral blouse can be worn sepa-

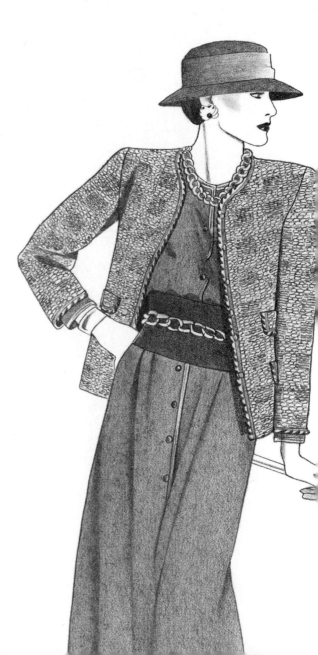

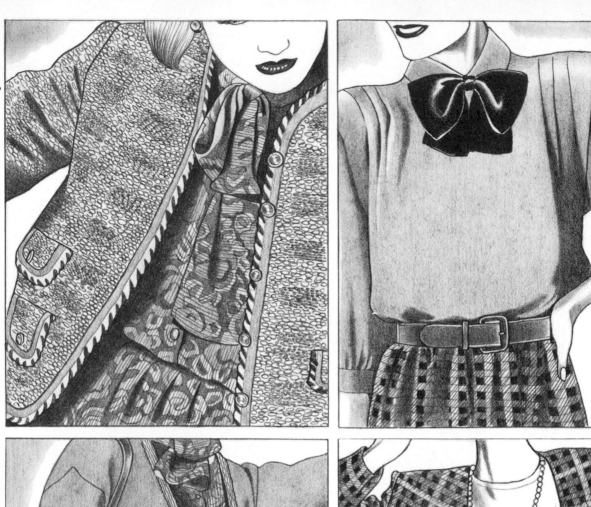
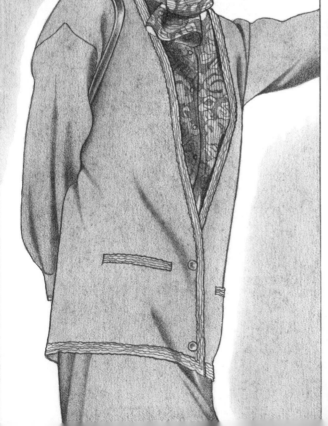
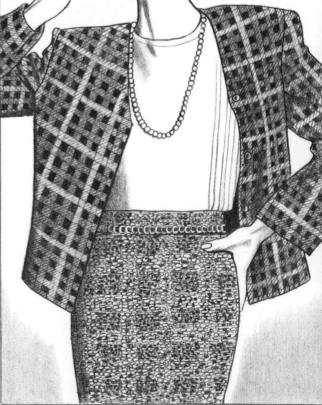

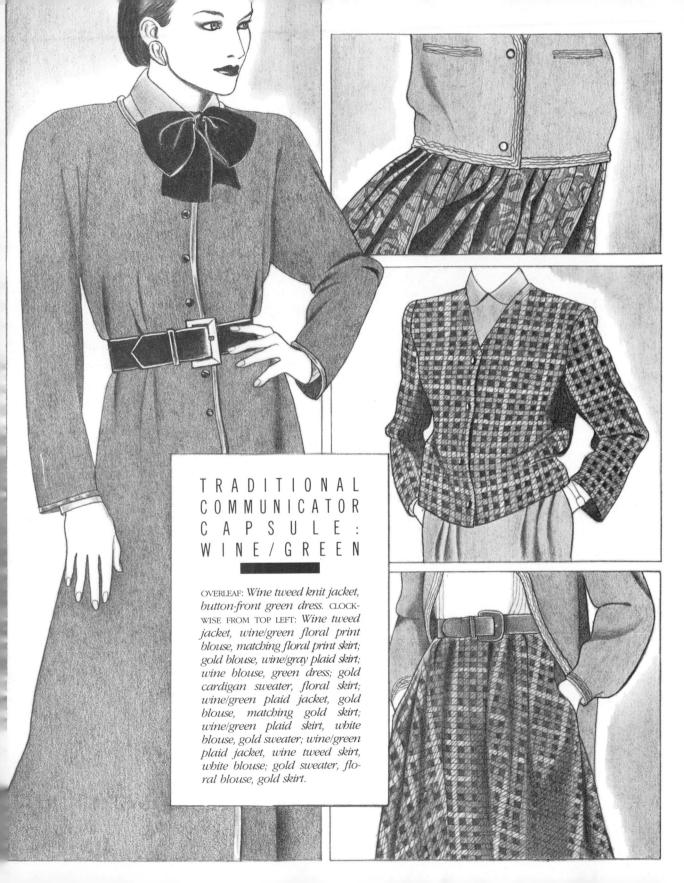

T R A D I T I O N A L
C O M M U N I C A T O R
C A P S U L E :
W I N E / G R E E N

OVERLEAF: *Wine tweed knit jacket, button-front green dress.* CLOCK-WISE FROM TOP LEFT: *Wine tweed jacket, wine/green floral print blouse, matching floral print skirt; gold blouse, wine/gray plaid skirt; wine blouse, green dress; gold cardigan sweater, floral skirt; wine/green plaid jacket, gold blouse, matching gold skirt; wine/green plaid skirt, white blouse, gold sweater; wine/green plaid jacket, wine tweed skirt, white blouse; gold sweater, floral blouse, gold skirt.*

rately with either the wine skirt or the plaid skirt, and the floral skirt can be teamed with either jacket and any of the blouses that are included.

A two-piece dress in the gold color works the same as the floral outfit. It too can be worn on its own or with either of the jackets. The blouse and skirt can also be thought of as separate components, to be combined in many different ways with the other pieces in the Capsule.

To give more color interest include one green dress. This is in a jewel neck, button-front style with gold button trim. Naturally, this dress too can be worn alone or with the jackets.

Besides the floral blouse and the gold blouse, there are two other long-sleeve blouses in this Capsule. One is in white, in a jewel neck, back-button style. The other is in wine in a soft shirt style with a detachable bow.

The last piece in this Capsule is a cardigan sweater. It is in the accent color of gold, and like the cardigan jacket, it has a braided edge that also uses the Capsule colors of wine and green. This sweater can be worn with any of the outfits to make a sophisticated yet casual look.

The twelve pieces in this Communicator Capsule are:

- ☐ Wine tweed cardigan jacket
- ☐ Wine tweed slim skirt
- ☐ Wine and green plaid jacket
- ☐ Wine and green plaid skirt
- ☐ Wine and green floral blouse
- ☐ Wine and green floral skirt
- ☐ Gold blouse
- ☐ Gold skirt
- ☐ White blouse
- ☐ Wine blouse
- ☐ Green dress
- ☐ Gold cardigan sweater

In combinations, they provide a varied, versatile working wardrobe for two months.

The second Communicator Capsule is based on *navy and white* in a variety of knit and woven looks including jackets, skirts, blouses and dresses. It is an excellent choice for travel as well as for daily dressing. The twelve pieces in the Capsule include *two jackets, one dress, three skirts, four blouses and two sweaters.*

A suit look is as important for the Communicator as it is for the Corporate woman, but the suit itself can be softer. In this Capsule we include two suit looks that are appropriate for meetings at any professional level. The suits may be made by Anne Klein II, Betty Hanson, David Hayes or Ernst Strauss. The first component is a navy knit jacket trimmed with white piping. We chose a matching navy knit skirt in a flat hip-stitched pleated style. Together they make a smart looking suit which can be worn easily from breakfast through dinner. The dark color dresses up the outfit and gives it an elegance that is appropriate for conferences or cocktails.

A second suit look is in white. If you live in a cold climate, you might not ordinarily wear white all year round. Fashion designers often show winter whites in their collections. Slightly softer and not as stark, these ivory shades give a fresh look to a dark wardrobe and may perk you up when you are tired of all the somber colors around. For this Capsule we'll use a white knit cardigan jacket that has a jewel neckline and patch pockets. The matching white knit skirt is a slim style. Of course, this makes an excellent suit look. You can also wear the navy blazer jacket with the white slim skirt and the white cardigan jacket with the navy

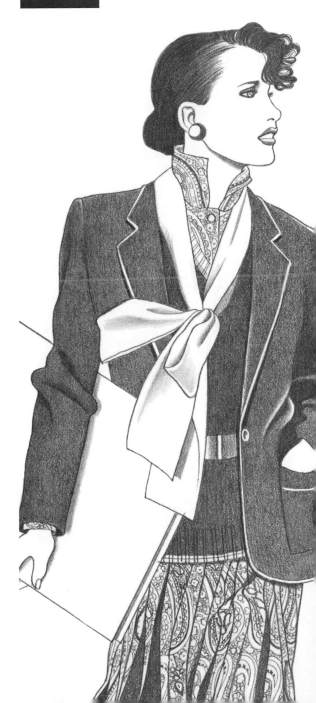

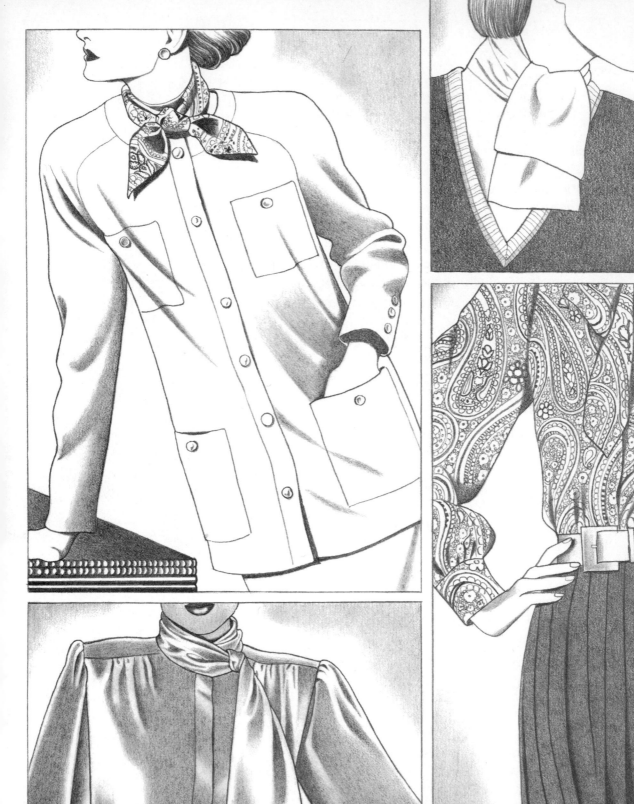

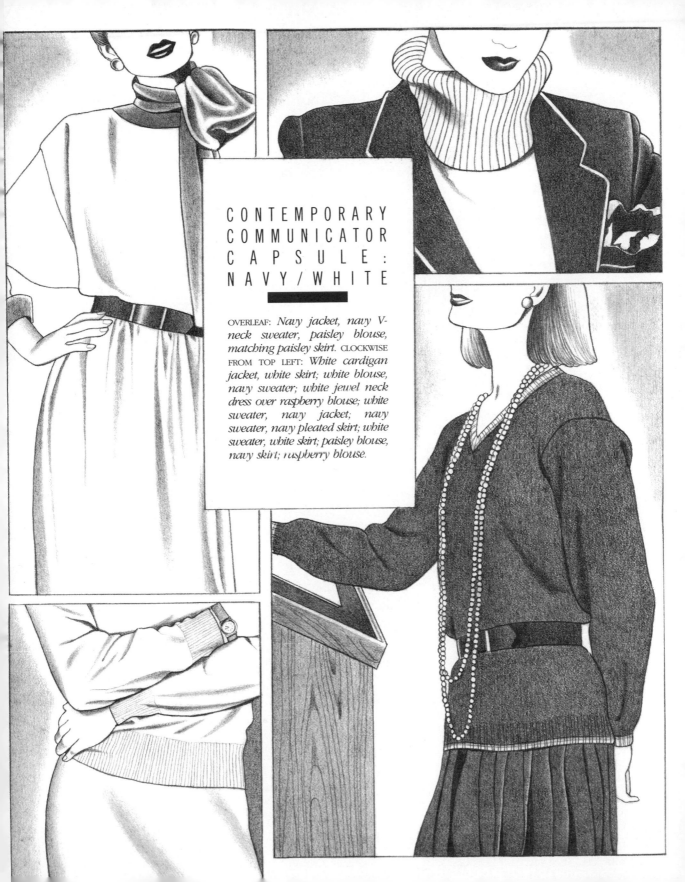

CONTEMPORARY COMMUNICATOR CAPSULE: NAVY/WHITE

OVERLEAF: *Navy jacket, navy V-neck sweater, paisley blouse, matching paisley skirt.* CLOCKWISE FROM TOP LEFT: *White cardigan jacket, white skirt; white blouse, navy sweater; white jewel neck dress over raspberry blouse; white sweater, navy jacket; navy sweater, navy pleated skirt; white sweater, white skirt; paisley blouse, navy skirt; raspberry blouse.*

pleated skirt. To give these outfits more of a coordinated, ensemble look, use a navy and white striped scarf around the neck, or a navy and white patterned blouse or sweater.

We also include a dress in this Capsule. The dress, in a white knit, is a jewel neck, long-sleeve style that can be worn on its own, with the white jacket for another complete suit look, or with the navy jacket for a contrasting dress and jacket look. The dress can also be worn with a blouse or sweater underneath it.

There is a second dress look in this Capsule but it is made by combining separates. These pieces may be from Evan Picone, Liz Claiborne, David Hayes or Jaeger. For this outfit we use a navy and white paisley printed silk blouse in a soft shirt style with a detachable bow and a matching pleated silk skirt. Worn together, these components make an elegant dress, once again appropriate for the office and afterwards. To give the paisley dress a more businesslike look, cover it with the navy knit jacket or the white knit cardigan jacket. The paisley blouse and skirt can also be worn as separates. For example, the paisley blouse works with the navy skirt or the white skirt and either of the jackets. The paisley skirt can be worn with those jackets and other blouses and sweaters. A matching blouse and skirt is one of the most practical and versatile ways to build different looks in your Capsule. It is also a good way to begin a Capsule. If you are not sure what colors or pieces to include in your wardrobe, start with a matching patterned blouse and skirt. Choose colors from that pattern to form the base of your Capsule, and select other blouses, skirts and jackets that work with it.

The three other long-sleeve blouses that we use include one white and two colors. Look for blouses that come with detachable scarves or bows and that have versatile necklines. You'll find that you can get many more looks from these styles; although they may cost more money, they're well worth the investment. The white blouse has a detachable stock tie and can certainly be worn with any of the skirts and jackets as well as with the navy dress. We then chose one blouse in a bright raspberry shade—one of the colors that is included in the paisley print. This blouse has a jewel neckline and its own separate scarf. The third blouse is in navy and it is in a shirt style with a convertible collar.

This Capsule has two sweaters. The first is a V-neck pullover in navy with white trim. It makes a coordinated look with either the navy knit pleated skirt or the white knit slim skirt. Both of these outfits look finished, yet relaxed and not as structured as a suit look. The pullover sweater can also be worn with the paisley skirt for a more casual style. The second sweater is a turtleneck in white, perfect to wear with any of the skirts and under the navy knit dress.

The twelve components in this Communicator Capsule give you looks that go from suits to casually coordinated, a range that most Communicators will find useful and practical. The pieces are:

- ☐ Navy knit jacket
- ☐ Navy pleated skirt
- ☐ White knit cardigan jacket
- ☐ White knit slim skirt
- ☐ White knit dress
- ☐ Navy and white paisley blouse
- ☐ Navy and white paisley skirt
- ☐ White blouse
- ☐ Raspberry blouse
- ☐ Navy blouse
- ☐ Navy pullover
- ☐ White turtleneck sweater

These twelve items give you forty different outfits for two months of different looks.

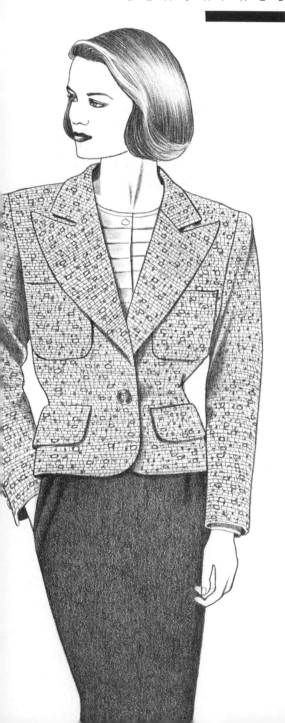

CONTEMPORARY COMMUNICATOR CAPSULE : BLACK/RED

The third Capsule for the Communicator woman is based on *black and red*. It also has suit looks and coordinated separates, from dressed up to dressed down, and includes *two jackets, four skirts, five blouses and one sweater*.

Because the Communicator can wear more relaxed styles, the suits in this Capsule are different from the others we have seen. They may be from designers such as Valentino or Ralph Lauren, or from more moderately priced firms such as Evan Picone or Ellen Tracy. The first jacket is in a black and gray tweed, with the peaked lapel jacket stopping at the hip. The matching tweed skirt is in a soft full style. This suit has the kind of flair that sends a message of vitality to the audience.

The second jacket is in red. It is single-breasted with a black velvet chesterfield collar and black button trim. To go with this jacket, we use a black slim skirt. This red and black combination makes another smart suit look that has an interesting twist to it. You can make more coordinated suit looks by putting the short tweed jacket with the black slim skirt and the red chesterfield jacket with the full tweed skirt.

This Capsule has a tartan plaid blouse in black, red, green and yellow, in a shirt style with a detachable bow. There is a matching tartan plaid pleated skirt. Together they make a striking dress which can be worn as it is, as well as with the tweed jacket or the red jacket.

Another dress look can be made with a matching solid red blouse that has its own black velvet bow, and a matching red dirndl skirt. It too can be worn by itself, and with the tweed jacket or the red jacket. These pieces may be from Pendleton, Evan Picone, Liz Claiborne or Spitalnick.

Think of both of the matching skirt and blouse outfits—the tartan plaid and the solid red—as separate components as well as dresses. The tartan plaid blouse can be worn with the tweed skirt, the black skirt and the red skirt along with either the tweed jacket or the red jacket. In a like manner, the tartan plaid skirt can be teamed with either of the jackets and any of the blouses that we will add to the Capsule. The solid red blouse can also be worn with the tweed skirt, the black skirt, and the tartan skirt along with the two jackets. The solid red skirt goes with the tweed jacket or the red jacket, and with all of the blouses.

This Capsule includes all long-sleeve blouses, one in white and two others in colors. The white blouse has a flat collar and covered placket closing. The colored blouses are one in black in a bow style, and one in yellow in a pleated front shirt style. All three of these blouses go with all of the skirts and can be teamed with any of the jackets. In the future, you might build a second Capsule around the tartan plaid, using the green and yellow as your base colors.

The last piece in this Capsule is a black sweater. Choose a long cardigan style in a thick knit that gives the authority of a jacket but the relaxed attitude of a knit. It goes with any of the skirts and blouses and even makes a suit look with the black skirt.

The snappy colors and happy plaids of this Capsule give you a bright, friendly look. The suits add a serious side that's right for corporate meetings and presentations. The components are:

- ☐ Black and gray tweed jacket
- ☐ Black and gray tweed skirt
- ☐ Red jacket
- ☐ Black skirt
- ☐ Tartan plaid blouse
- ☐ Tartan plaid skirt
- ☐ Red blouse
- ☐ Red skirt
- ☐ White blouse
- ☐ Black blouse
- ☐ Yellow blouse
- ☐ Black sweater

These twelve pieces make enough outfits for three working months.

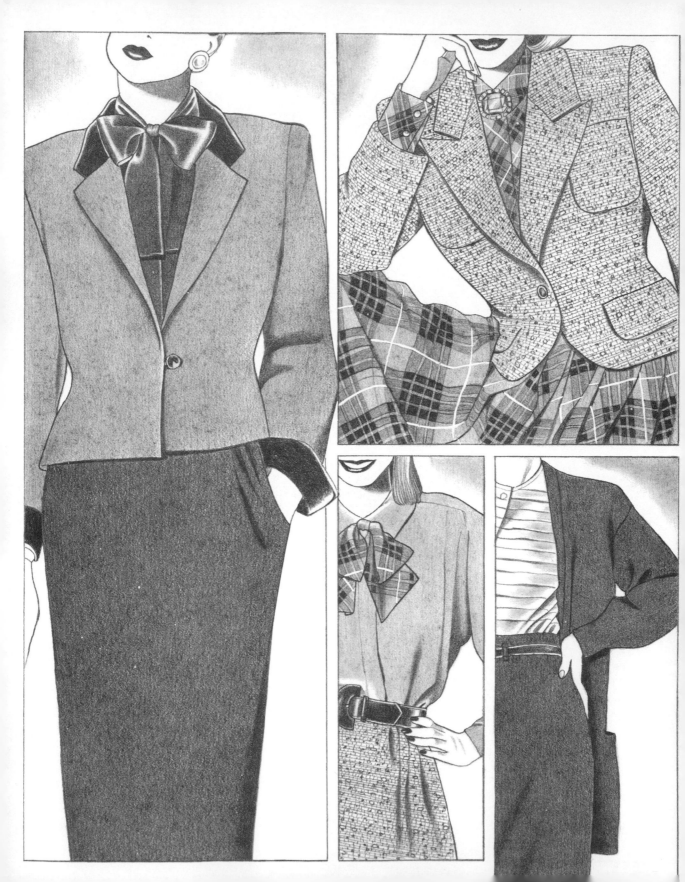

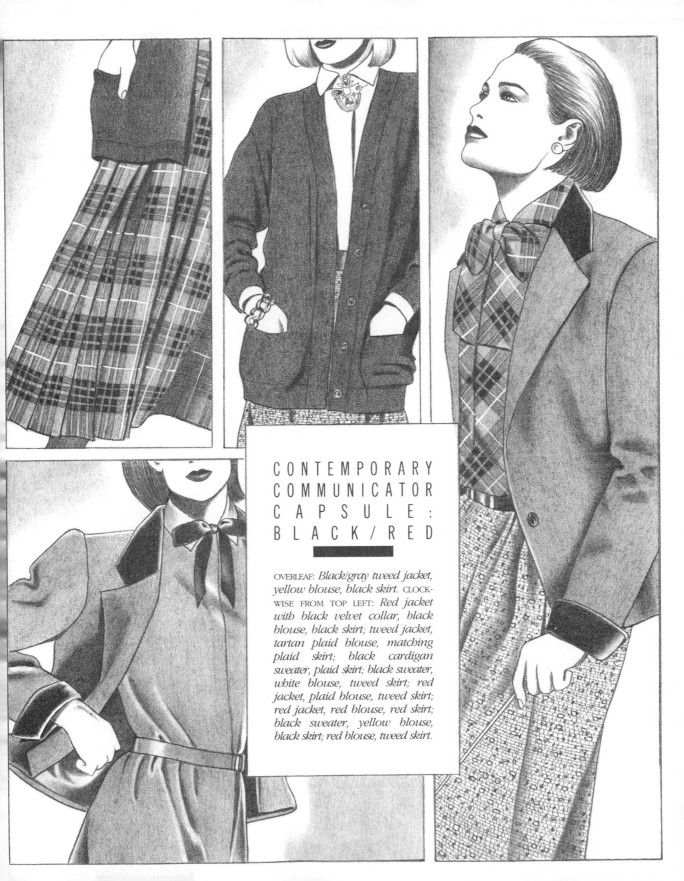

CONTEMPORARY COMMUNICATOR CAPSULE: BLACK/RED

OVERLEAF: *Black/gray tweed jacket, yellow blouse, black skirt.* CLOCKWISE FROM TOP LEFT: *Red jacket with black velvet collar, black blouse, black skirt; tweed jacket, tartan plaid blouse, matching plaid skirt; black cardigan sweater, plaid skirt; black sweater, white blouse, tweed skirt; red jacket, plaid blouse, tweed skirt; red jacket, red blouse, red skirt; black sweater, yellow blouse, black skirt; red blouse, tweed skirt.*

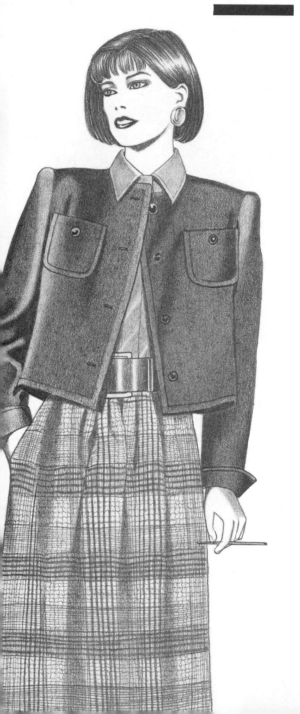

The fourth Communicator Capsule is more innovative and places an emphasis on textures. The colors are *black and cocoa* and the fabrics incorporate a mix of soft mohairs and crisp tweeds, plush suedes and lush silks. There are *two jackets, three skirts, one pair of pants, one dress, four blouses and one sweater*.

To begin this tactile Capsule we'll start with a buttersoft cardigan style jacket in black suede. This jacket represents the major investment in the Capsule, but it produces a striking return. Lightweight suedes are now available that can be worn all year round, and they look dressy or casual depending upon how you treat the outfit. They may be private label imports or carry designer labels such as Blassport or Calvin Klein.

The next component is a full dirndl skirt done in a black and cocoa plaid. The skirt can be combined with the black suede jacket for a coordinated yet casual suit look.

There is also a black and cocoa plaid in an asymmetric buttoned jacket in the same fabric as the dirndl skirt. This outfit produces a proper matched suit look, although again, because of the pattern and style, it is more relaxed than the typical matched Corporate suit.

A second skirt is in black and cocoa tweed in a box pleat style. Because the colors are the same, this skirt can be worn with the plaid jacket for an interesting mix of texture and pattern, a look done by Escada and David Hayes. This same tweed skirt also looks excellent with the black suede jacket.

The innovative Communicator can sometimes include pants as well as skirts in her Capsule. In this case we use a pair of black trousers. If you do include pants in your Capsule, bear in mind that the most businesslike pants are in crisp fabrics such as gabardine or flannel, and in dark colors such as black or navy. They look most appropriate for work when they are worn with a matching jacket. The black suede jacket provides the polished, finishing touch to this ensemble. Of course, the pants can be worn with the black and cocoa plaid jacket, although this has a casual look. To give the plaid jacket and black pants a more finished look, use a black blouse with it, or a white or cocoa blouse with a black bow at the neck.

We use one true dress in this Capsule, a black knit in a long-sleeve, button-front, jewel neck, slim skirt style. This type of dress is smart and crisp looking on its own, and looks great with the black and cocoa plaid jacket or the black suede cardigan jacket. This dress can also be worn over the blouses that follow.

A second dress look comes by combining a soft wool jersey shirt in cocoa with a matching full soft skirt. As with the black dress, it looks perfectly appropriate on its own, or when worn with the asymmetric plaid jacket or with the black suede cardigan. These jersey components, however, can also be treated as separates. The shirt goes with the black and cocoa plaid dirndl skirt, with the black and cocoa tweed skirt, and with the black trousers. Either of the jackets can be worn on top. The cocoa jersey skirt can be combined with the jackets as well as with the blouses that are included.

In this Capsule there are four long-sleeve blouses, including the cocoa jersey shirt. As always, one of the blouses is white. No matter if your Capsule is Corporate or Communicator, classic or casual, at least one white blouse is essential. It adds a crispness and gives you the kind of versatility that is so important to long-term investment dressing. This particular blouse is a white silk shirt with a tuxedo front. A second blouse is in beige in a plain shirt style. The third blouse is in a rust color with a bow neckline. All of these blouses work with any of the skirts and pants and can be topped by either of the jackets. They are also worn under both the black dress and the cocoa dress.

The last piece in this Capsule is a mohair sweater in a multi-colored patterned cardigan that includes black, cocoa and rust. The sweater adds a rich finishing touch to any of the skirts, the pants, or the two dress looks.

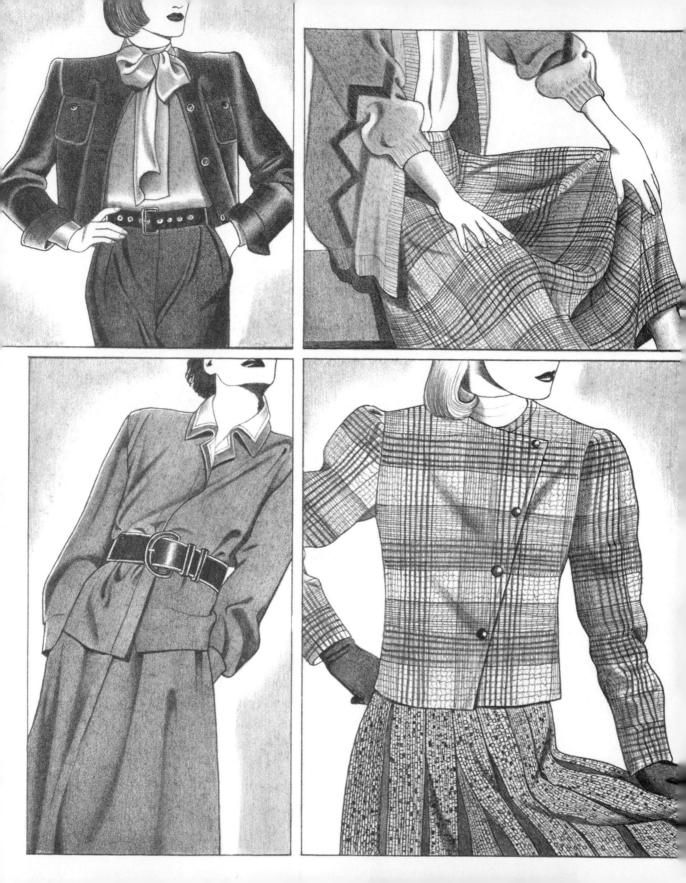

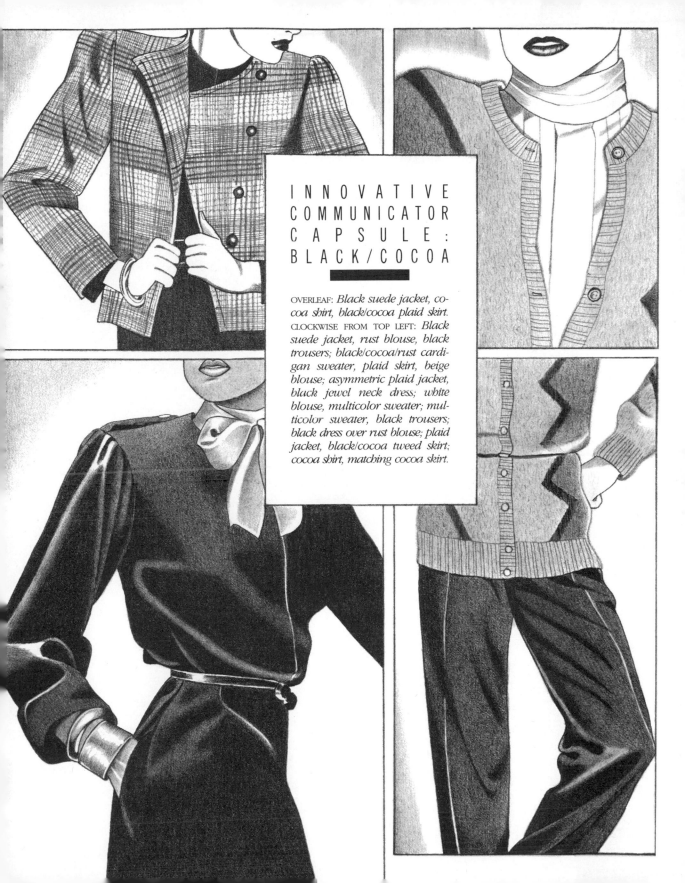

INNOVATIVE COMMUNICATOR CAPSULE: BLACK/COCOA

OVERLEAF: *Black suede jacket, cocoa shirt, black/cocoa plaid skirt.*
CLOCKWISE FROM TOP LEFT: *Black suede jacket, rust blouse, black trousers; black/cocoa/rust cardigan sweater, plaid skirt, beige blouse; asymmetric plaid jacket, black jewel neck dress; white blouse, multicolor sweater; multicolor sweater, black trousers; black dress over rust blouse; plaid jacket, black/cocoa tweed skirt; cocoa shirt, matching cocoa skirt.*

The twelve pieces in this Communicator Capsule give you a broad range of looks. The components are:

- ☐ Black suede jacket
- ☐ Black and cocoa plaid asymmetric jacket
- ☐ Black and cocoa plaid skirt
- ☐ Black and cocoa tweed skirt
- ☐ Black trousers
- ☐ Black button-front dress
- ☐ Cocoa jersey shirt
- ☐ Cocoa jersey skirt
- ☐ White blouse
- ☐ Beige blouse
- ☐ Rust blouse
- ☐ Multicolor sweater

Once again there are forty looks to take you through eight working weeks.

ACCESSORIES FOR THE COMMUNICATOR CAPSULE

Accessories are a valuable tool for the Communicator. They act as a focal point or conversation piece, and make it easy for someone to approach you and begin to talk. Choose bright colors and bold pieces.

A small group of components can serve you well: two pairs of shoes, one handbag, two belts, three scarves, two pairs of earrings and two necklaces. You may decide to add some extra pieces, but use these as your base.

The first Capsule is in wine and green. Both colors work with all of your clothes. The wine is neutral enough so that you may choose it for both pairs of shoes, but by selecting two different colors, you can create a much more varied effect. When picking two different colors, select both in the same style, or select one in a plain pump and the other in a slightly different look. In the second Communicator Capsule, the colors are navy and white. Since white is a limited color, I suggest using navy for both pairs of shoes in this Capsule. Choose two different styles so that you can get a varied look with your outfits. For example, select one pair of pumps and one slingback style or some other version of a classic look—such as a patent tip, a walking shoe or a spectator style. The third Capsule is based on black and red. Black shoes are an excellent choice for serious meetings and conferences. A pair of red shoes can add excitement and flavor to your wardrobe, but be careful to stay with a simple style. The not-so-traditional color is enough; don't overdo it. In the fourth Communicator Capsule, the color combination is black and cocoa. Since both of these are neutral colors, they are both good colors for your shoes.

The color of your handbag also coordinates with your Capsule and helps to give you a neat, tidy and precise look. But you might choose a more expressive style, such as a pouch, a large shoulder bag, or, if you carry papers but don't want an attaché, a large leather envelope. There are wonderful handbags on the market for women who carry more than their keys, wallet and checkbook, but don't want the look of a real briefcase. The first Capsule, in wine and green, can take either color handbag. Generally, wine is an elegant and neutral shade which can work well with other Capsules as you build, so it may be the preferable color. For the navy and white Capsule, choose a navy bag. It goes with all of your clothes and works year round. If your Capsule is black and red, you may select either color. The black is more serious and dressy, the red fun and easy-going. The black and cocoa Capsule lends itself to a handbag in either color too. Again, the black is the dressier color, better if you tend to go out often after work.

If you carry an attaché, briefcase or portfolio, look for one that is feminine in feeling. A heavy or mannish case can be intimidating; a more feminine one can still look efficient but have some fashion to it. Just as the Corporate woman, be sure to select a handbag—envelope, clutch or small shoulder bag—that can fit inside your attaché. A woman who struggles with shoulder bags and briefcases tends to look like a bellboy rather than a businesswoman. Portfolios and attachés come in colors like wine, attractive tans, and even bright reds which give them some style and take away from the heavy, masculine look.

The other leather items in your Capsule are your belts. These are also in the Capsule colors and help give your outfits a finished, complete look. The basic styles are always safe and sure—about an inch and a half wide with a plain buckle will work with all of your clothes. However, some of the Communicator Capsules can take a more un-usual belt. Rather than plain leather, consider suedes or skins such as lizard, alligator or even eel. They give a more interesting, textured look but can still be in basic styles. You might choose a wider leather sash and a bold accent color for a second belt.

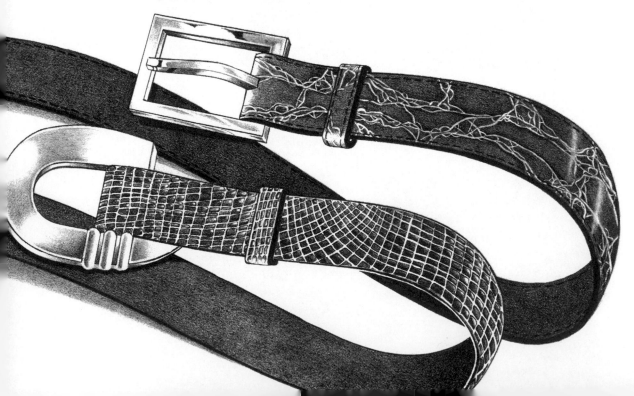

Scarves are an excellent way to bring in other colors, add fashion, and change the look of your clothes. While the Corporate woman must be fairly conservative, as a Communicator, you can have more fun. Stay with natural fibers such as silk or fine wool because scarves are a worthwhile investment. The oblong styles are still the most versatile, but look at fashion magazines to learn the latest way to tie a scarf. If your blouses come with detachable bows so that you already have your Capsule colors covered in your neckwear, look for other solids or interesting prints that pick up your colors and include some others in the patterns.

The Communicator can use jewelry that brings an outfit together and adds some interesting features. For example, choose earrings and necklaces in pearl, gold or silver, but look for hammered gold or hand-made silver styles. You might consider oversized earrings or delicate antiques. Jewelry is a wonderful accessory to begin collecting; it's an excellent investment and it can provide an easy conversation point.

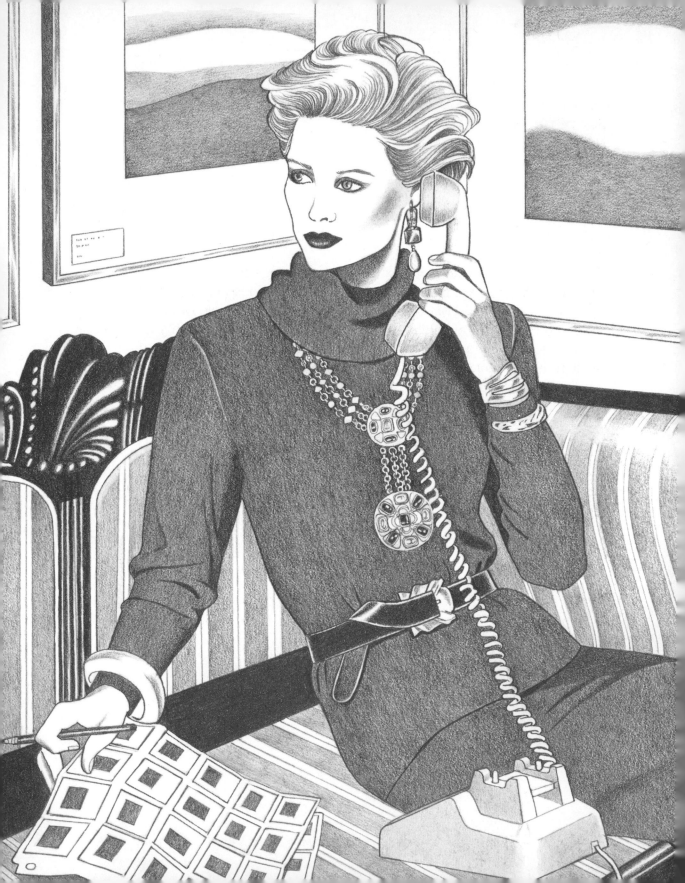

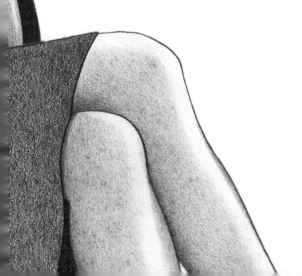

CHAPTER VIII

The Creative Capsule

To the Creative woman, clothing is more than a tool, it is an art form, a means of expression. The body is a blank canvas on which to work. The Creative woman thinks in terms of the way colors relate, the way textures interplay, the way shapes take form, and the final work becomes a whole.

The Creative woman chooses colors the way an artist does; she experiments with the palette of colors, choosing pale pinks, soft blues, gentle yellows. She may work boldly with gossamer fabrics such as fine jerseys, light crepes, wafer-thin cottons and handkerchief linens, with yet more verve applying rich reds, royal blues, shocking pinks, neon greens and brilliant yellows to her canvas. Or she may equally well experiment with mysterious blacks, midnight blues, poppy reds, marigold yellows, foggy grays and oyster whites. She can be bold or subtle and very unpredictable; she wears her moods and interests on her back.

There are movements too, and time frames: the elegance of Edwardian dressing, the striking contrasts of the Color School of painting, the minimalism of the moderns. With her Creative touch she may follow a group or go out on her own, but whichever way she chooses, she has her own stamp and style, her mark of identity.

In a way it may be unfair to suggest a Capsule for the Creative woman. It is her ability to be imaginative that gives her the freedom to select her own clothes. But there are many women who may use these Capsule ideas as a taking-off point, a way of beginning a wardrobe in this direction. I have seen several women move from staid, traditional styles of dressing to strong, innovative looks. By watching, reading and experimenting, they learned how to play with clothes, how to make their clothes work for them, and how to make their clothes express their individuality. Sometimes they started with one or two pieces which they added to their wardrobes. After enjoying them and learning how to adapt them to the rest of their clothes, they have gone on to add more and more experimental looks. You may decide to do the same. Invest in one or two pieces, perhaps a special handknit jacket or supple suede skirt, and see how it adds uniqueness to your wardrobe.

Creative Capsules are also perfect for traveling. If you're planning a trip, and want to get away from your Corporate or Communicator profile, this is the place to do it. These relaxed clothes are easy to pack, take up little room, and give you dozens of different looks. It's also fun to experiment when you're away from home, so think about using these ideas for your next getaway.

The three Capsules in this chapter range from innovative to avant-garde. You'll see how to work around several different looks, from spare, pared-down dressing to layers of color and cloth. Like the Capsules in the other chapters, they each have twelve basic components based on two colors, with all of the pieces interrelated. By experimenting with new and different combinations, the number of outfits that you can make from them is almost endless.

The Creative woman has the luxury of being able to wear almost any color, any texture and any shape. Choose your palette to suit your taste and your moods. It might be strong one day and pale the next. You need not worry about matched suits or simple lines. Rather, contrast solids, mix patterns, and enjoy the freedom of unconstructed clothes. If you favor simplicity, create a monochromatic scheme of angled lines. Look for clothes of the highest quality, clothes that give you a long term return on your investment. Fashions change, but style doesn't.

The first Creative Capsule is based on *black and white*. To it we add some shocks of accent colors, hot pink and royal blue. The pieces in the Capsule are all in knits. They include *one jacket, two pairs of pants, two skirts, three dresses and four tops.* These clothes may come from Calvin Klein, Anne Klein or Donna Karan. In particular, Donna Karan believes that black is a basic color for any wardrobe and bases her collection on building around a Capsule of fundamental pieces.

The knit jacket is a simple style, long-sleeved, collarless and hip length that may be from Perry Ellis or Adrienne Vittadini. The only patterned piece in the group, it is in a striking, multicolored pattern that picks up all of the colors in the Capsule, including the accent shades. It can be worn alone, buttoned, or over any of the tops and dresses.

The first pair of pants are in black and are cut with narrow legs. Naturally, they work with the patterned jacket and any of the tops. The second pair of pants are in white. This time we use a more classic, straight-leg style. Again, they go with the patterned jacket, although the look is quite different.

We chose two different shapes for the skirts, again one in black and the other in white. The black skirt is shorter and straight, while the white skirt is long and soft. Both skirts are worn with the patterned jacket.

The first sweater is a long-sleeve, black turtleneck, perfect with the black pants or black skirt for a long narrow look, or with the white pants or white skirt for a sharp contrast. It can be tucked in or worn

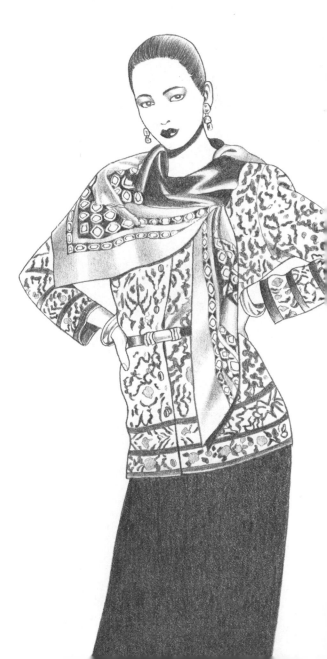

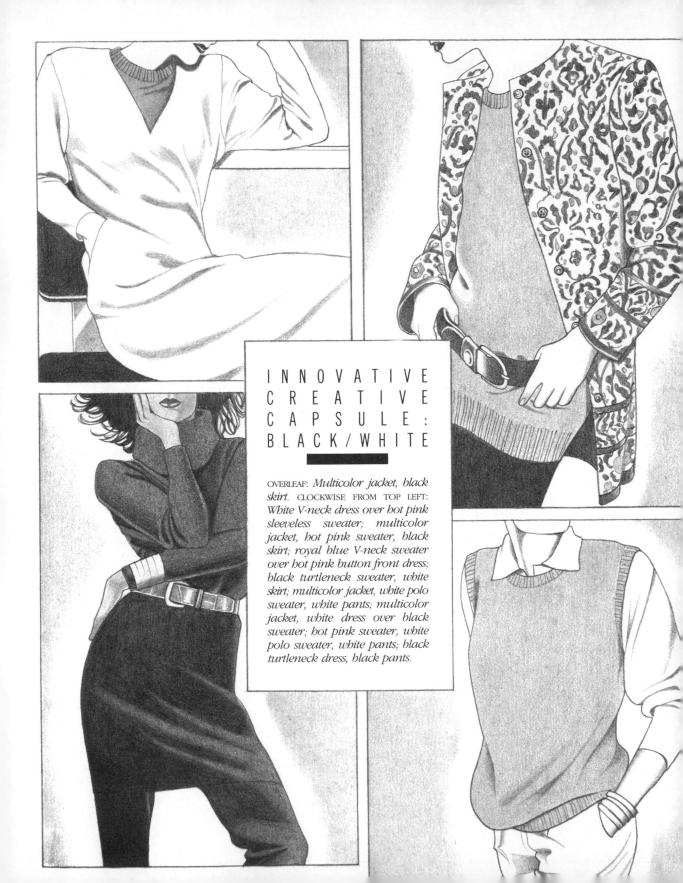

INNOVATIVE CREATIVE CAPSULE: BLACK/WHITE

OVERLEAF: *Multicolor jacket, black skirt.* CLOCKWISE FROM TOP LEFT: *White V-neck dress over hot pink sleeveless sweater; multicolor jacket, hot pink sweater, black skirt; royal blue V-neck sweater over hot pink button front dress; black turtleneck sweater, white skirt; multicolor jacket, white polo sweater, white pants; multicolor jacket, white dress over black sweater; hot pink sweater, white polo sweater, white pants; black turtleneck dress, black pants.*

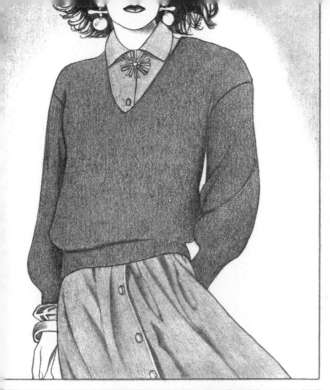
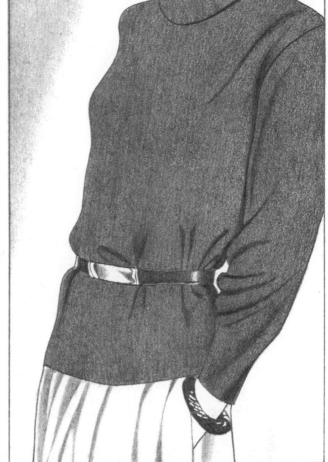
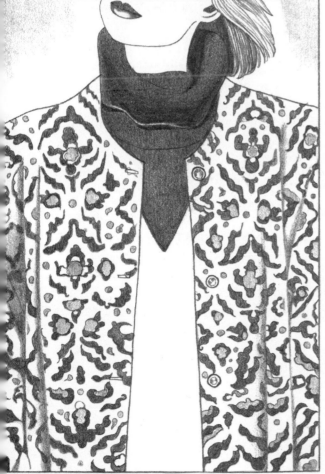
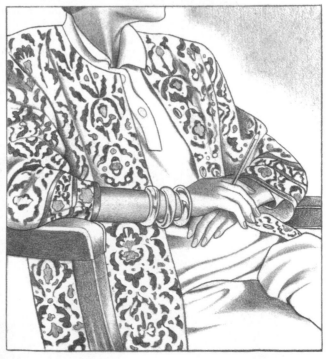

out, tunic style, belted or not. It can also be worn under the patterned jacket.

The second sweater is a white polo shirt style with placket front and long sleeves. It too can be tucked in or worn out, with a belt or without, and can also be worn with the turtleneck underneath. It works with the black pants, the white pants, the black skirt and the white skirt.

The third sweater is a round neck, sleeveless style in an accent color of hot pink. It works with the black pants, the white pants, the black skirt or the white skirt. This sleeveless top can be worn alone as well as over the turtleneck or the polo shirt. And it can be worn under the multicolored jacket.

The fourth sweater is a V-neck style with long sleeves in the accent color of royal blue. Like the others, it goes with either the black pants or the white pants, and the black skirt or the white skirt. It can be worn in or out, as well as over the turtleneck and the polo shirt. It can be worn under or over the sleeveless round neck top, and also works with the patterned jacket. With these tops, you can create a pared-down look or a multilayered style.

The first dress is a black, long-sleeve, straight style with a large turtleneck. It can be worn as is, or belted, or as a tunic by wearing it over either of the pants or the skirts. It can take the white polo shirt or the black turtleneck underneath it, and the hot pink sleeveless sweater or the royal blue V-neck sweater over it. It can also be worn with or without the patterned jacket.

The second dress is a long-sleeve, V-neck style in white. Like the black dress it can be worn as a tunic over the black pants or skirt or the white pants or skirt. It can also be worn plain or belted. This dress works on its own, or over the black turtleneck sweater or the white polo sweater. Both the hot pink sleeveless sweater and the royal blue V-neck sweater can be worn over it or under it. It can be worn alone or covered up with the multicolored jacket.

The third dress is a button-front long-sleeve style in hot pink. It can be worn as a dress, a tunic or a coat. It can take any of the tops—the black turtleneck, the white polo shirt, the hot pink sleeveless or the royal blue V-neck—underneath. It can be paired with the black pants, the white pants, the black skirt and the white skirt, and can also be worn with the patterned jacket.

This Capsule of monotones and color blocks includes:

- ☐ Multicolor patterned jacket
- ☐ Black pants
- ☐ White pants
- ☐ Black skirt
- ☐ White skirt
- ☐ Black turtleneck sweater
- ☐ White polo sweater
- ☐ Hot pink sleeveless sweater
- ☐ Royal blue V-neck sweater
- ☐ Black turtleneck dress
- ☐ White V-neck dress
- ☐ Hot pink button-front dress

The possibilities for these twelve pieces are almost endless. They can take you through months of work or travel. It's up to you to create as many different looks as you like.

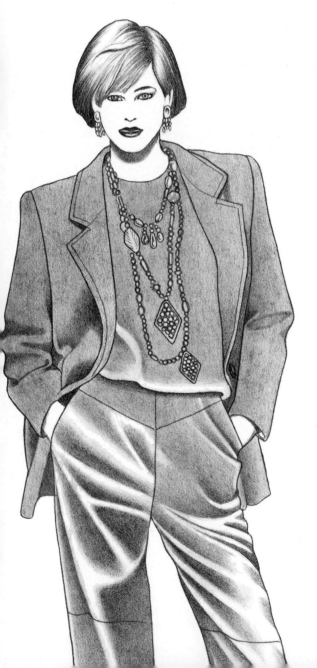

INNOVATIVE CREATIVE CAPSULE: CAMEL/CREAM

Let's take an entirely different approach with the second Capsule. This time we'll use a color combination of *camel and cream* for a mostly monochromatic effect. The emphasis, however, is on textures as we interplay rough and smooth, heavy and light, knit and woven. These clothes act as a perfect background for interesting accessories such as belts, scarves and jewelry. Like the first Creative Capsule, this is an excellent Capsule for travel, and even includes components that can double for work or play, often a necessity when traveling. The pieces include *two jackets, two pairs of pants, two skirts, three blouses, two sweaters and one dress.*

The first jacket in this Capsule is in a smooth camel's hair done in a double-breasted style. Although it has a classic look, which can be important for the Creative woman who is facing her Corporate or Communicator counterparts, it can also work as a sophisticated cover for any of the outfits in this group.

The second jacket is a cream-colored cardigan worked in a curly mohair that is soft yet has a very textured effect. It has no collar or buttons, and rounded shoulders, giving it a loose, easy look. These jackets and the pieces that follow may come from Ellen Tracy, St. Tropez West, Calvin Klein or Blassport.

There are two pairs of pants, both of them in classic shapes. The first pair is in a menswear trouser, fly front, pleated at the waist and cream-colored. The fabric is a soft flannel. This pair of pants works well with either the camel double-breasted blazer for a contrast look or with the cream mohair cardigan for a subtle pantsuit look. The second pair of pants are straight-legged in a soft tan leather that also goes well with either of the jackets, but creates a more casual look.

The two skirts again offer different fabrications and different styles. The first skirt is a long, A-line style in a rich shade of tan. It is done in a soft, supple suede that feels comfortable and moves easily. It can be worn with either the camel jacket or the curly mohair jacket. The second skirt is a soft wool, long, dirndl style in a camel and cream herringbone. Naturally, it goes with the camel's hair as well as the curly mohair jacket.

The dress in this group is a knit jersey in a cream color. It has a jewel neckline, long sleeves, and a long, full, flowing skirt. It can be worn alone, pared-down, or perhaps with one bold belt or decorated with a smashing scarf or jewelry. It can also be topped with either the camel jacket or the cream jacket. The dress, the pants and the skirts can all be worn with the tops that follow.

There are three blouses in this innovative Creative Capsule. The first is an ivory silk, long-sleeved, double-breasted shirt style. Its collar can be worn in different ways, up or down, buttoned or unbuttoned. Like the camel jacket, it is classic and the perfect backdrop for special accessories such as necklaces, pins or scarves.

The second blouse is a simple, thin suede top with a jewel neck, button back and long sleeves. It's in the same tan shade as the suede skirt. It can be worn outside, belted or not, or tucked into the suede skirt or the tweed skirt, and with the leather pants or the trousers. When worn with the suede skirt, it has the effect of a dress.

The third blouse is in a cream color in a silky charmeuse fabric. It has a pointed shirt collar which can be worn open or closed and full dolman sleeves that give it a dramatic effect. It goes with both pairs of pants and both skirts. This blouse can also be worn under the jersey dress, or can double as a jacket and go over any of the tops.

We added two sweaters to this Capsule. The first one is a turtleneck style in a beige cashmere. It is worn with the cream menswear pants or the camel leather pants, and with the tan suede skirt or the tweed skirt. It is also worn under any of the blouses and under the dress. Both jackets work well over it.

The second sweater is a very textured, oversized cowl neck, long-sleeve style done in a mix of yarns both shiny and dull and in all shades of creams and camels. It is excellent with both pairs of pants and both

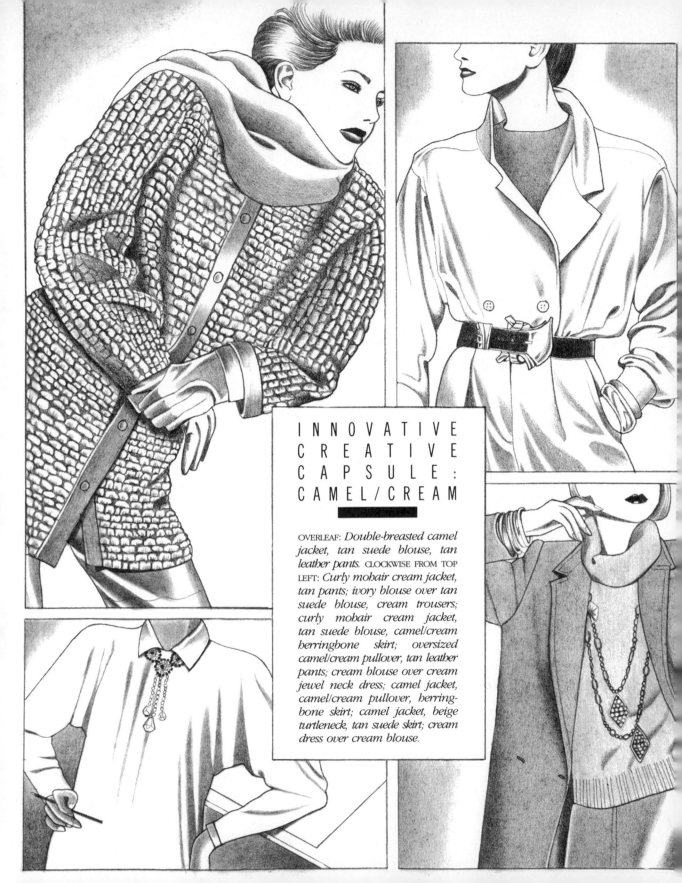

INNOVATIVE CREATIVE CAPSULE: CAMEL/CREAM

OVERLEAF: *Double-breasted camel jacket, tan suede blouse, tan leather pants.* CLOCKWISE FROM TOP LEFT: *Curly mohair cream jacket, tan pants; ivory blouse over tan suede blouse, cream trousers; curly mohair cream jacket, tan suede blouse, camel/cream herringbone skirt; oversized camel/cream pullover, tan leather pants; cream blouse over cream jewel neck dress; camel jacket, camel/cream pullover, herringbone skirt; camel jacket, beige turtleneck, tan suede skirt; cream dress over cream blouse.*

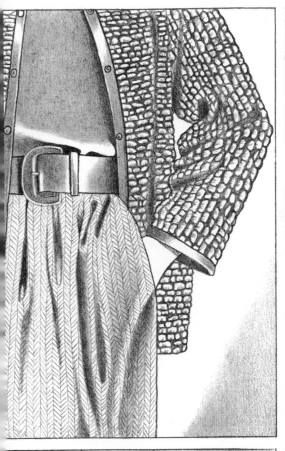

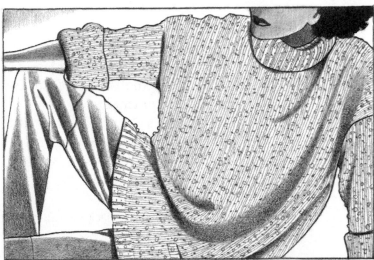

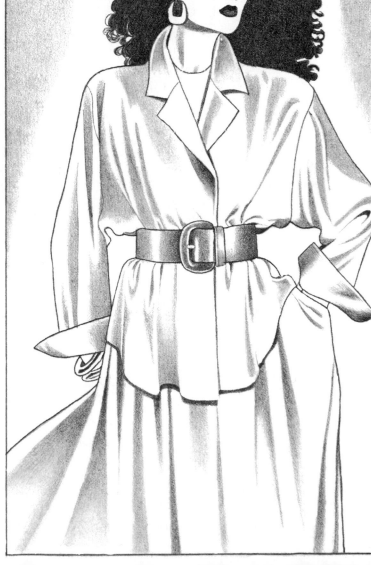

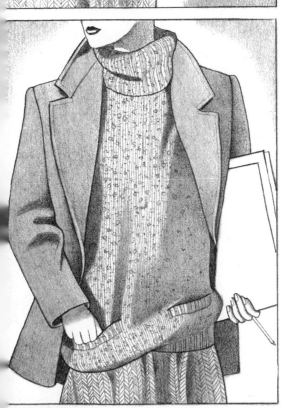

skirts, and can be worn over or under the dress. This sweater also looks stunning with either the camel jacket or the cream jacket.

With its emphasis on texture and monochromatic colors, this Creative Capsule includes:

- ☐ Camel's hair double-breasted jacket
- ☐ Curly mohair cream jacket
- ☐ Cream trousers
- ☐ Tan leather pants
- ☐ Tan suede skirt
- ☐ Camel and cream herringbone skirt
- ☐ Cream jersey dress
- ☐ Ivory silk blouse
- ☐ Tan suede blouse
- ☐ Cream blouse
- ☐ Beige turtleneck sweater
- ☐ Camel and cream cowl neck sweater

Remember that these twelve pieces may be particularly good for travel.

The third Capsule emphasizes shape, going from long, narrow lines to soft, well-rounded ones. The two basic colors of the Capsule are *mustard and black,* but there are strong accents of red and purple. The components in this group are *two jackets, two pairs of pants, two skirts, one blouse and five sweaters.* These are the kinds of clothes that may come from Perry Ellis or Claude Montana.

The first jacket is in mustard in a sweeping cocoon style with wide shoulders and raglan sleeves coming down to a narrow hemline below the hip.

The second jacket is in an accent color of red. With epaulets and brass buttons, square shoulders and straight lines, its angular shape is very different from the rounded mustard jacket. It may be from a new designer collection or found in a thrift shop.

There are two pairs of pants in this Creative Capsule and once again, they are very different. The first is a dark mustard jodhpur style, with soft pleating at the waist, rounded at the hips and then straight-legged from the knees down. Combined with the mustard jacket, it has a soft, sculptural style. When teamed with the red jacket, it has the look of a riding habit.

The second pair of pants, in black, are very skinny from waist to ankle, in perfect contrast to the jodhpurs. They too can be teamed with either jacket, composing very different effects.

This Capsule has a long, slightly flared skirt in the mustard color. We chose a jersey fabric with a soft flowing look. This skirt too can be worn with either jacket.

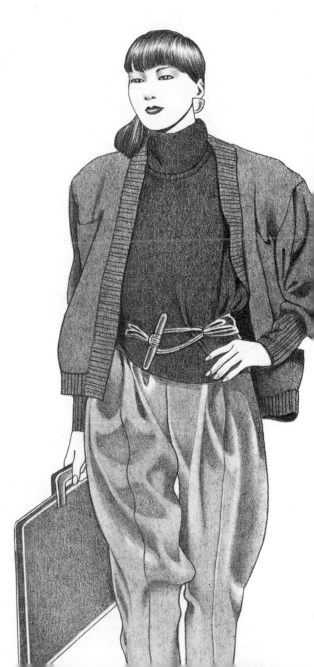

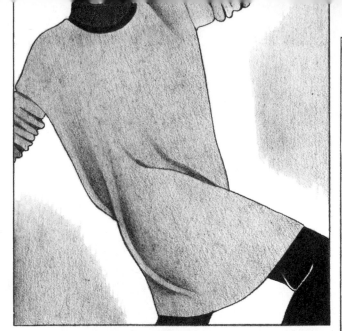

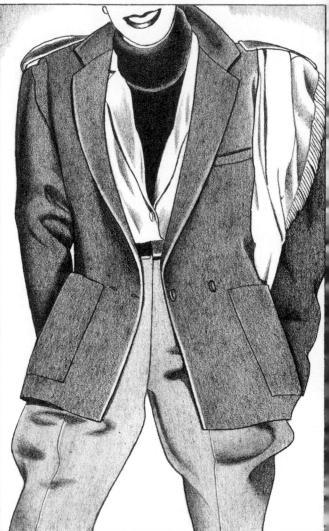

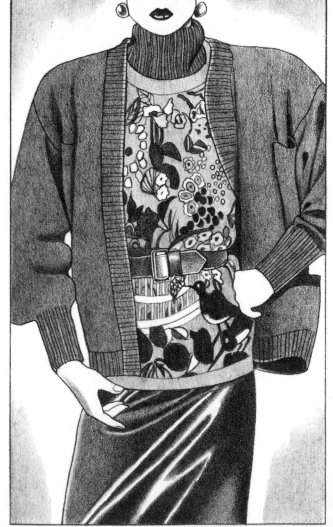

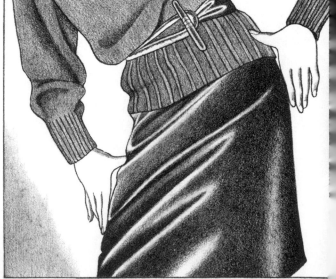

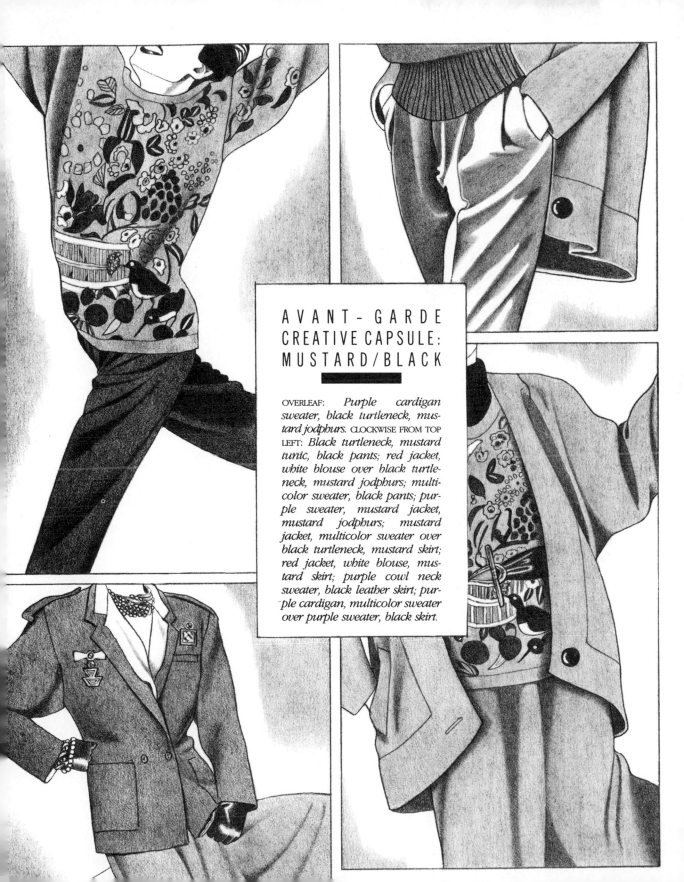

AVANT-GARDE CREATIVE CAPSULE: MUSTARD/BLACK

OVERLEAF: *Purple cardigan sweater, black turtleneck, mustard jodphurs.* CLOCKWISE FROM TOP LEFT: *Black turtleneck, mustard tunic, black pants; red jacket, white blouse over black turtleneck, mustard jodphurs; multicolor sweater, black pants; purple sweater, mustard jacket, mustard jodphurs; mustard jacket, multicolor sweater over black turtleneck, mustard skirt; red jacket, white blouse, mustard skirt; purple cowl neck sweater, black leather skirt; purple cardigan, multicolor sweater over purple sweater, black skirt.*

The second skirt is a straight style in soft black leather. It too goes with both the red jacket and the mustard jacket. This skirt has more of a sharp, angular look to it than the softer jersey skirt. Any of the tops goes with it.

There is only one blouse in this Capsule. It is a long-sleeve white silk shirt with a convertible collar. It can be worn simply as a plain shirt or accessorized with jewelry and scarves. Tuck the shirt into the jodhpurs or the black pants, or wear it outside the black pants like a poet's tunic. It also goes with the long mustard skirt and with the straight black skirt. Naturally, either jacket works well over it.

There are five sweaters in this Capsule, each a different style and shape. The first is a mustard color tunic with a round neck and long sleeves. It is combined with the mustard skirt to create the look of a dress, worn with either pair of pants, on its own, or over the white blouse. The tunic works well with either jacket.

The second sweater is a black turtleneck. It too goes with the black pants, the jodhpurs, the mustard skirt or the black leather skirt. It can be worn alone, under the white blouse, or under the mustard tunic. Both jackets work with it.

The next two sweaters are in the second accent color, purple. One is a cowl neck long-sleeve style. It is worn inside or out of both pairs of pants and both skirts. It also goes under the white blouse or the mustard tunic. This cowl neck style goes under either the red jacket or the mustard one. The other purple sweater is a blouson cardigan, again giving round lines to the overall picture. It can be matched with the cowl neck pullover for a sophisticated sweater-set look, or worn over the blouse or the other sweaters. The cardigan can be belted and worn underneath the jackets.

The last sweater is a scooped neck, patterned pullover that picks up all of the colors—the mustard, the black, the red and the purple. Naturally, it goes with all of the pants and skirts and works well under the jackets. The solid color sweaters and blouse are also worn under it.

The twelve pieces in this Capsule are:

- ☐ Mustard cocoon jacket
- ☐ Red jacket
- ☐ Mustard jodhpurs
- ☐ Black skinny pants
- ☐ Mustard jersey skirt
- ☐ Black leather skirt

- [ ] White silk blouse
- [ ] Mustard tunic
- [ ] Black turtleneck sweater
- [ ] Purple cowl neck pullover
- [ ] Purple blouson cardigan
- [ ] Multicolor pullover

These pieces create a variety of shapes and looks, ranging from serious to amusing, business to weekend wear.

ACCESSORIES FOR THE CREATIVE CAPSULE

The Creative woman has the opportunity to indulge in the most unusual accessories. They are another way of expressing imagination and inventiveness. You may find pieces in flea markets or thrift shops, in art galleries or crafts shows, or you may even make them yourself.

Two pairs of shoes are a good starting point for your accessories Capsule. The styles that you choose as basics may be as classic as Anne Klein pumps in alligator or lizard, or something more adventurous like multicolor suedes from Maud Frizon or Charles Jourdan. If you attend meetings with your colleagues in the corporate world, take that into consideration. One pair of closed shoes may be a good investment. Yves Saint Laurent and Pancaldi make forward fashion styles that are not outrageous. On a more moderate scale, so do Perry Ellis, Beenebag, and Joan and David.

Handbags too can be very imaginative. Look for interesting textures, unusual shapes or bold color combinations. In a Capsule of black and white, for instance, choose a multicolored handbag. Belts also allow for creativity. Look for odd shapes, unusual materials and bold clasps. An interior designer I know scouts antique shops and buys old clasps, pins, and even tops of cigarette cases, which she then turns into belt buckles.

When you are selecting scarves, look for several different shapes. There are large shawls, long oblongs and big squares that can all be used to enhance your outfits. Turn a plain jersey dress into something smashing by wearing a beautiful, patterned shawl over one shoulder or a striped scarf wrapped around the waist. An oversized bow worn under the collar of a blouse makes an ordinary shirt into something very special. A sweater and pants become chic with the twist of a muffler. Or tie two scarves together for another interesting effect.

The jewelry that you use can be quite unusual and helps identify you as a Creative woman. It you invest a lot of money in one piece, make it your signature. For instance, Carrie Donovan, fashion editor for the *New York Times Magazine,* is known for her rows of bangles on her arm. Other women wear loads of chains or choose one individual piece that really stands out. It can be a serious piece of jewelry or an amusing fashion item. At an antique show not too long ago, I found a costume pin, oversized and filled with "rubies, emeralds and diamonds." I have worn it on strands of pearls or pinned it to a dress and it gives a dramatic look. People look twice, not sure if it's real or fake. When you're building a Creative Capsule, you can indulge in whimsy, having fun with your clothes and your accessories.

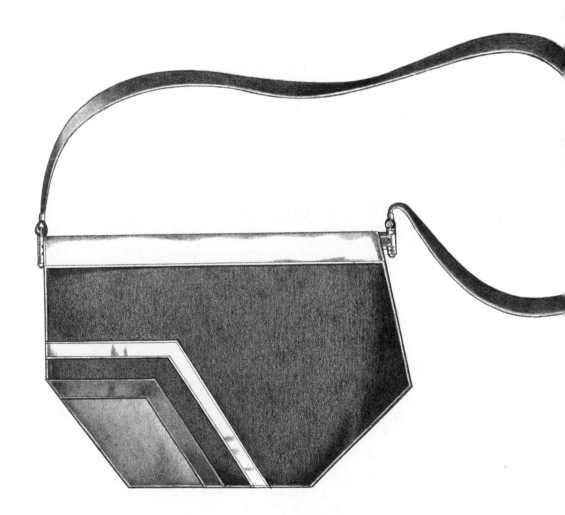

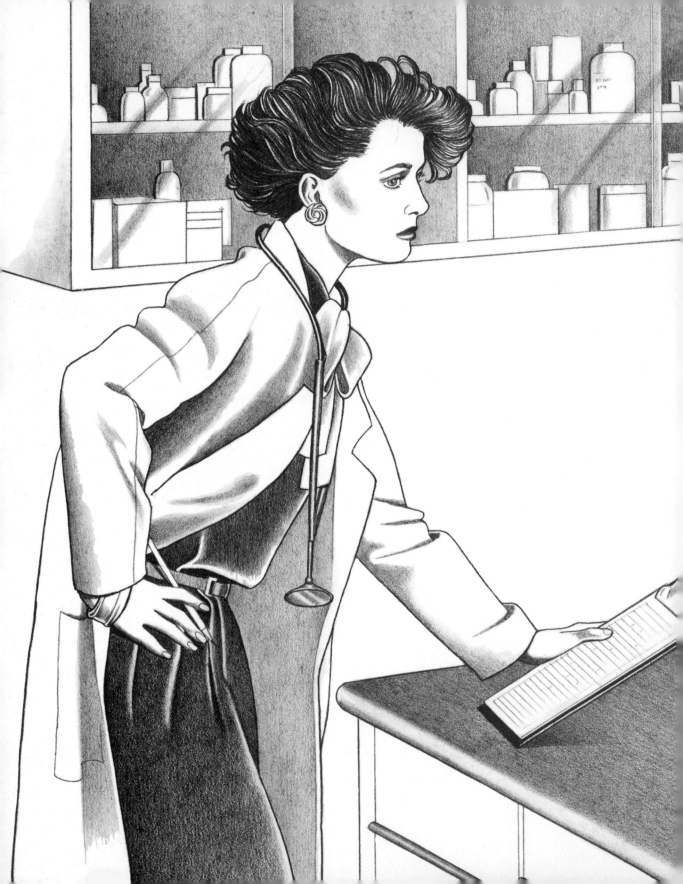

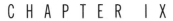

Real Uniforms: Career Service Profile

Millions of women work at jobs that aren't included in the Corporate, Communicator or Creative profiles. This fourth category, called Career Service, may apply to you if your work requires wearing a true uniform and if it entails taking care of people. For instance, if you're in the field of health or beauty care, work for an airline or in certain sales organizations, you are in a Career Service area. With over three million people in the health care field alone, this profile encompasses a large proportion of working women.

Our clothes talk about us, as we know, and wearing a uniform says a great deal about who you are. Career apparel, which is another way of saying "uniform," is the visually distinguishing mark of Career Service. It works as an identity tag for your audience, which consists of those you're helping, those who are your peers, and those who are above you on the career ladder. The uniform distinguishes you from the rest of the crowd and sets you apart from them. At the same time, it links you with the rest of your team. In a hospital, in a doctor's office, on an airplane, and even in an office or retail outlet, there can be confusion over who is in charge. The uniform immediately identifies you as a member of the professional team, as a person to be called upon for help.

If you wear a uniform, you probably already know the advantages. Not only does it enhance your position and give you authority, it also makes wardrobe building easy. It eliminates the ordeal of putting new outfits together every day or worrying about the latest looks in fashion. Shopping is simplified, dressing is effortless, and your closet isn't cluttered with unnecessary clothes.

But there are liabilities as well. Career apparel can become boring if you're faced with the same colors and styles day in and day out. It may be harder for the outsider to distinguish you from your colleagues because you all look alike. And you may be spending so much of your clothing budget on career apparel that you have little left over for your leisure wardrobe.

There are several ways of focusing on your appearance so that your uniform still allows you a certain amount of individuality. The uniform styles you choose, the accessories you put with it, your hairstyle and your makeup all help to form your overall appearance. Given two people of equal ability, the one who looks crisper and more efficient is more likely to get ahead. If you look organized, people assume you are organized. If you look as though you respect yourself, others respect you too. If you look attractive, those you are caring for and those you are working with respond positively to you, which, in turn, gives you an even better feeling about yourself.

Judith Goldstein is a pediatrician in New York City. The mothers who come to her office are mostly working women, and she sees herself as a role model for them. Underneath her white lab coat the petite doctor wears sophisticated clothes. She feels her sense of identity is strengthened by her attractive appearance.

When she started her practice ten years ago, she was concerned that her interest in fashion might undermine her credibility. Instead she quickly saw that the women who came to her liked her clothes sense, could identify with it and even found it inspirational. "I see a lot of women. Women want someone to admire, a role model to guide them for the future. If you work fourteen hours a day you feel better if you're dressed up. I also find that good clothes maintain their look and hold up well."

Says five-foot, three-inch Dr. Goldstein, "I am a Nipon addict." Albert Nipon dresses are perfect for her size four figure. She bases her Nipon choices on fashion ideas she picks up shopping the Yves Saint Laurent boutiques. Because she wears a white lab coat so much of the time she believes, "You lose your sense of identity unless you maintain your sense of fashion."

Like this elegant doctor, you can probably enhance your appearance with some fashion touches. Wear smart clothes under your uniform, or choose interesting accessories or jewelry to wear with it. Not everyone can afford to buy dresses by Albert Nipon, but there are contemporary clothes at every price point. Chaus, Koret, Jones, Liz Claiborne and others make separates and dresses that you might consider.

Although uniform styles are fairly conservative and limited, there is usually enough of a choice to offer you a variety of looks in your wardrobe. Dresses, tops, skirts and pants are available in different silhouettes. It will boost your morale to vary the styles in your uniform selections. Look for different necklines such as jewel necks, V-necks, mandarins and shirt collars. Include different fabrications (even polyester comes in a variety of textures) such as woven linens, crepes, gabardines, broadcloths, and knits in your wardrobe. Look for different details, such as embroidery, pleats, shirring, smocking, piping and pockets as well as short sleeves, long sleeves, raglan sleeves and set-in styles, and choose different colors if they are allowed. In the field of health care, you may be permitted to wear whites and pastels like pink, blue and yellow. As an airline flight attendant, you may be offered solids and prints; if so, choose both so that you can create different looks. Select a variety of styles—in skirts choose wraps, button fronts, side closings and culottes. Add pants and jumpsuits to your wardrobe as well. In dresses, choose different designs such as step-ins, shirtwaists, zip fronts, back buttoned and jumper styles.

Career Services profiles who are limited to wearing whites and pastels may consider the use of cardigan sweaters. Most health care workers are permitted to wear sweaters in pastels, navy and other colors as well. That touch of color breaks the monotony, enhances the look of your clothes, and gives you a more dynamic presence.

Jewelry can also help give you a positive image. Although jewelry should be kept to a minimum, you may consider earrings as an attractive addition. Styles which sit on the ear are best; small hoops, balls, knots, shells and geometrics are all available in gold or silver. Use some color here as well. A necklace can also highlight an outfit. Try a single strand of pearls, a small pendant or even colored beads. Pins are another way of enhancing your uniform. Like earrings or necklaces, they give your audience something to focus on besides your clothing. A pin that is amusing can relax your listener or encourage a sense of camaraderie. A pretty pin can be a conversation point as well as a way of making your uniform more attractive.

Perhaps more than anything else, good grooming is essential. In fields that require orderliness and authority, a crisp, efficient appearance says that your work habits are the same way. It gives your audience confidence in you. It says that you pay attention to details, that you are in control and someone who can be trusted to do the job well. A fresh, clean uniform and polished shoes are essential.

Since most uniforms are made of machine washable synthetics, cleanliness should not be a problem, especially if you own interchangeable components. You can build a Career Apparel Capsule that gives you maximum looks and minimum investment with ten to twelve pieces. Choose at least two dresses, two skirts, one pair of pants and five tops for a variety of looks. If you own a pantsuit or a two-piece dress, separate the tops and bottoms and count them as two pieces. Treat them as separates and wear them with other parts of your Capsule. Hang them separately in your closet so that you will not think they are locked in as outfits. Since you wear these clothes every day and your professional image relies on them, you owe it to yourself to have enough styles to give you a feeling of change from day to day.

Your makeup and hairstyle can enhance your attractiveness and help you to look more efficient. You don't need much makeup to give you polish. Choose cosmetics that give you a natural, fresh look. Anything heavy will take away from your look of competence and detract from your professionalism.

Just as your makeup should help you look noteworthy without being noticeable, your hair should flatter your face without being the focus of your audience's attention. Clean, glossy hair sends a message that you are competent and care about yourself. Hairstyles that are below shoulder length, that are frizzy or teased or fall in your eyes should be avoided. If you have long hair, wear it off your face, and keep it in place with barrettes, a rubber band, or combs. This type of look gives you yet another opportunity to brighten up your appearance with some color. If you use a rubber band, finish it off with a bright-colored ribbon, or choose barrettes or combs in pretty colors. If you like to wear your hair loose, keep it no longer than chin length and hold it in place with a hairspray that isn't stiff.

If you dress in a uniform all week, take advantage of leisure clothes to add fun and color to your wardrobe. Many nurses have told me that they have little money left over from their uniform purchases for their weekend or evening wardrobes. They spend their free time in a warmup suit or jeans and a T-shirt. But this doesn't give them the opportunity to express themselves through their clothes or even to enjoy dressing. You can do this without spending a great deal of money if you build a Leisure Capsule. With a small wardrobe of twelve clothing components based around two colors you can have a multiplicity of looks that will take you from casual dates to special occasions.

The key to this Leisure Capsule is using color. If you wear white or pastels during the week, choose strong colors for your own time. For example, work around a Capsule of navy and yellow, red and black, or purple and pink. Add accent colors so that your wardrobe is not limited. This is the one place where a splash of color is almost a necessity; it gives you extra vitality and energy. When selecting accent colors, think again in terms of colors that go together. You may be able to build a second Capsule with two of your accent shades.

Although you may immediately want to go for high-styled clothes, save these for later or pick up fashion trends in your accessories. Start with classic shapes and you'll find they last longer and give you more flexibility. These are the components that will work for you for looks that range from casual to dressy.

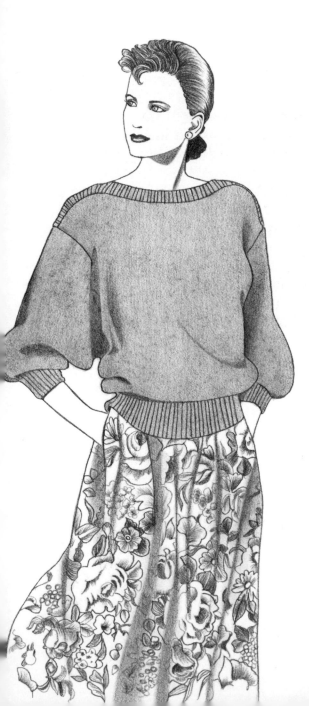

As an example of a Leisure Capsule, we'll work around *navy and rose*. The pieces include *two pairs of pants, two skirts, three blouses, four sweaters and a jacket.* If you spend most of your working time in dresses or skirts and like to wear pants, leisure time is when to do it. A solid pair of pants in a dark color, such as navy, black or gray, can look relaxed or regal depending upon what you wear with it. As a guideline, choose dark colors if you want dressy looks that can also double for casual wear. In this case we use navy pants. Choose a second pair of pants in another color to give you a change of pace. For instance, introduce an accent color of purple and pick pants in that shade. Purple pants might sound bold, but remember that this is your chance to have fun with your clothes. There should be at least two skirts in this Capsule as well, and here again use two different styles. The first skirt is a rose one in a straight silhouette. The second skirt is in a softer style in a print. Let's use a floral pattern that combines navy, rose, purple and yellow, although you can as easily choose a geometric or a plaid with the same colors. Now you have four different bottoms and may select tops that work with all of them.

For the first top, select a rose blouse in the same shade as the rose skirt. It is in a silky fabric and has a convertible collar that can be worn open or closed. This blouse goes with the navy pants, the purple pants and the floral skirt, and for an added plus it can be combined with the rose skirt to look like a dress. This means that you'll be able to create casual as well as more dressed-up looks with it. A second top is a navy blouse in a shirt style that has a detachable bow. It also goes with the four bottoms. This navy blouse looks very dressy when worn with the navy pants, particularly if we use the bow and add pearls to the outfit. The third blouse is in the floral print that matches the patterned skirt. Together they make a dress that can be worn for many different occasions. The print blouse also goes with the two pairs of pants and the rose skirt.

This Leisure Capsule includes several sweaters as they too can swing from casual to special occasion. The first sweater is a pullover in rose. It can be worn alone with any of the skirts and pants, or over the yellow, the rose, the navy and the print blouses. The second sweater is a purple turtleneck. It too can be worn on its own with the navy pants, the purple pants, the rose skirt or the floral skirt, and it can also be worn under any of the blouses or the rose sweater. The third sweater is a yellow cowl neck that brightens everything in your Leisure wardrobe. It goes with the navy pants, the purple pants, the rose skirt or the floral print skirt. The last sweater is a bold stripe of navy, yellow, purple and rose in a thick knit cardigan style. It goes with any of the solid color bottoms and makes an interesting combination with the floral skirt because the colors are the same.

The last piece is a jacket. Let's choose a rose cardigan style that coordinates with any of the skirts or pants and goes over any of the tops. For instance, wear the navy pants with the yellow sweater and the rose jacket for a very vivid look. Or combine the rose jacket with the matching rose skirt for a stunning suit. The rose jacket goes over the purple pants or the print skirt, and each time you'll be creating different looks and moods with your leisure clothes. The components include:

- ☐ Navy pants
- ☐ Purple pants
- ☐ Rose skirt
- ☐ Floral print skirt
- ☐ Rose blouse
- ☐ Navy blouse
- ☐ Floral print blouse
- ☐ Rose pullover
- ☐ Purple turtleneck sweater
- ☐ Yellow cowl neck sweater
- ☐ Bold stripe cardigan
- ☐ Rose cardigan jacket

These pieces can work for weekend and evening wear and for travel.

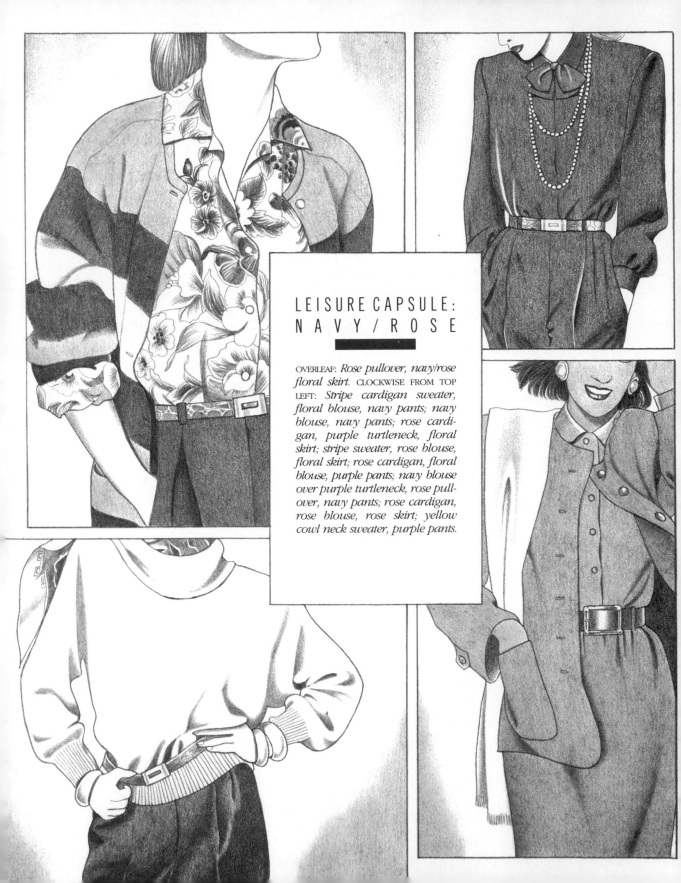

LEISURE CAPSULE: NAVY / ROSE

OVERLEAF: *Rose pullover, navy/rose floral skirt.* CLOCKWISE FROM TOP LEFT: *Stripe cardigan sweater, floral blouse, navy pants; navy blouse, navy pants; rose cardigan, purple turtleneck, floral skirt; stripe sweater, rose blouse, floral skirt; rose cardigan, floral blouse, purple pants; navy blouse over purple turtleneck, rose pullover, navy pants; rose cardigan, rose blouse, rose skirt; yellow cowl neck sweater, purple pants.*

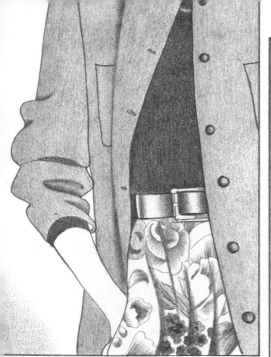
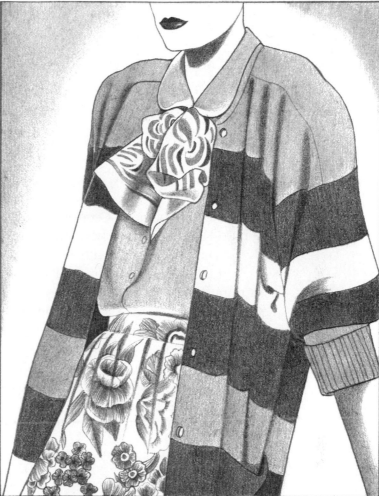
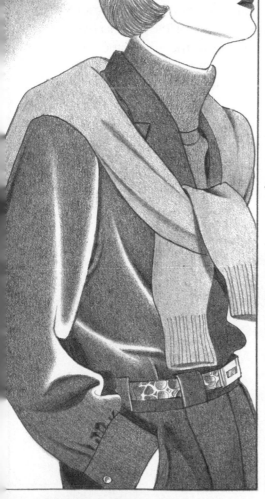
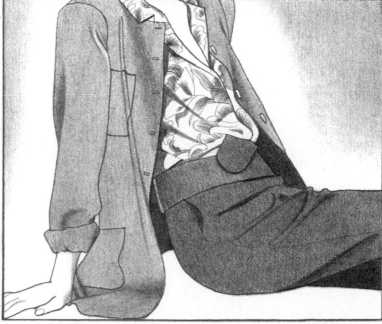

Finishing Touches

Whether you are a Corporate, Communicator or Creative woman, it's important to have the basic accessories you can rely on. They should go with all of the clothes in your Capsule, pull together your outfit, and give a finishing touch to your look. The right hosiery, earrings, watch and scarf can make a big difference. Recently I was a guest at a luncheon and fashion show for a new women's shop. The clothes were all expensive, all imported from Italy, styled by well-known designers and worn by professional models. The owner of the shop, however, had no understanding of accessories; the clothes looked flat. The well-dressed audience lost interest in the show and the owner lost potential customers. Don't lose *your* audience by looking so-so. Finish your statement with accessories, and top it off with the right coat.

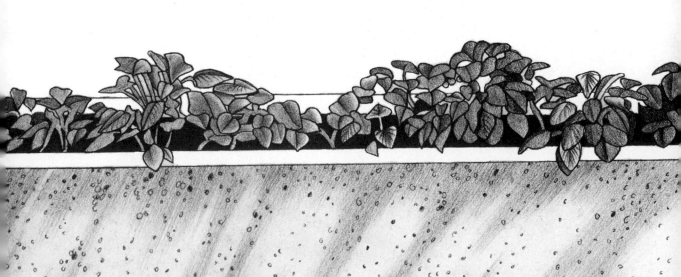

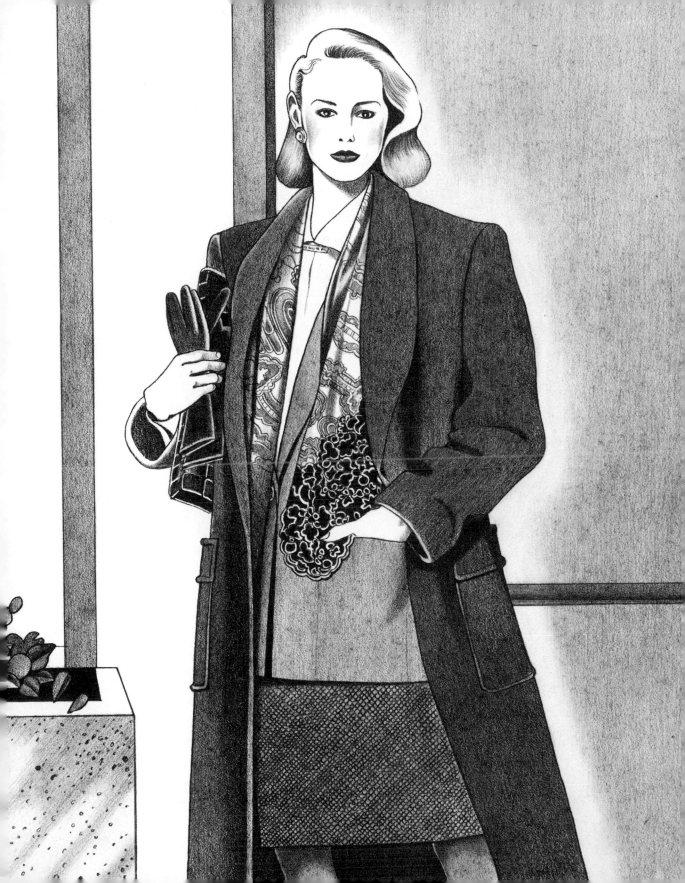

LEGWEAR. One of the least expensive and most effective ways to pull your outfit together is with hosiery. Fashion looks in legwear change from year to year, and by changing your hosiery you can update your look and give your clothes a whole new attitude. When putting together your wardrobe, spend a few minutes trying on different types of hosiery with your outfits and see how the looks vary. To get a long, lean look choose hose and shoes in the same color as your skirt. If your legs are heavy, dark colors make them appear slimmer. Conversely, light shades and textured hose help a too-thin look.

The Corporate woman should be fairly traditional in her legwear, but there are subtle changes that can update even a conservative wardrobe. For example, the most classic hosiery is a sheer, "nude" style. There are years, however, when color plays a more important fashion role, and the Corporate woman can use a tinted, sheer stocking for a more interesting and coordinated look.

Legwear can be used to tone down or dress up an outfit. The Communicator has more leeway and can use opaque or patterned styles when they are in fashion. Be careful, though, to stay away from looks that are overpowering. Subtle patterns are easier on the eye. Your audience may not be ready to accept stark white or bright red legs. On the other hand, colored hosiery can bring a whole outfit together.

The Creative woman can take advantage of all of the fashion looks in legwear. You may decide to use one style as your individual statement, always wearing black stockings or coordinating the color of your hosiery with your clothes. Or, you may stay closer to the current trends, whatever they may be. Even if your clothes are classic, an individualistic approach to your hosiery can help give you an innovative look.

When shopping for legwear, be aware of the importance of proportions. Generally, heavy, textured styles look best with low-heeled shoes. The lighter and paler the hose, the dressier the look will be. Lacey looks and ornamented stockings may be too delicate for everyday wear and are best left for evening or non-work times. Do check the fashion magazines and store displays to see what's new in legwear. Color and texture can make the difference in an outfit.

EARRINGS. Earrings add polish to your appearance. Like an exclamation point, they don't just finish a statement but give it punch. Try on different styles, sizes and materials to see how they can change the look of any outfit. Gold and pearls generally look richest and most elegant; bright colors add pizzazz; silver or ivory are sophisticated. To see how earrings affect an outfit, try a simple black dress with gold or pearls for a chic look, with bright red for a bold look, with silver for a sleek look.

With traditional and contemporary clothes, simple earclips are best. There's room for color, texture and interestings shapes, but keep to styles that stay close to the ear and don't interfere with your overall look. More innovative styles of dressing allow for more inventiveness in earrings. Nevertheless, remember that long, dangling styles are best for evening—they can be distracting for day. Have one or two basic styles in gold or silver that work with most of your clothes. That's a big help when you're rushing to dress or uncertain of what accessories to use with an outfit. You'll feel more comfortable knowing that you can count on these earrings to give a finishing touch to your outfit.

WATCHES. Watches have taken on social status and fashion identity. The Rolex, the Cartier Tank, and the Concord Mariner are all expensive status symbols. You may find it desirable to wear one of these styles as a symbol of your success, or you may want to avoid wearing them at any cost.

A watch is both a timepiece and a piece of jewelry. For best investment return, choose a style that can be worn for both day and evening. Leather, lizard, suede or alligator bands are all appropriate. Dark color bands in black, navy, brown or wine work with most outfits. A simple gold band can also work well yet give a dressier look. Be sure the numerals are clear and that you can read them easily. A few years ago I invested in a beautiful watch that had an abstract face. The watch had won a museum award for its design, yet I found it almost impossible to tell the time: I was constantly struggling to read it. No matter what style you choose, be sure that your watch keeps good time. Your timeliness is one clear mark of your efficiency.

SCARVES. No matter what your Profile, there are times when you'll want to use scarves for different effects. You can use almost any shape if you follow some simple directions for folding them. Refer to the illustrations as well on pages 192–193.

If you have a square scarf and want to use it as a triangle, lay the scarf flat on the angle of a diamond shape, and bring the top point to the bottom point. If you want to fold the square on the bias, then lay the square flat, as a diamond shape again, and fold the top and bottom points to meet in the center. Then continue folding them in towards the center. If you want to make the square into an oblong, lay it flat and fold the bottom side toward the center and the top side over it towards you. Continue to fold it like this until you reach the desired width. If you already have an oblong scarf and want to make it narrower, lay it flat and bring both long sides to the middle. Continue folding it in until you arrive at the width you want.

A long square scarf folded into the bias shape works for a dog collar or muffler look. Hold one end of the scarf in each hand and place the middle of the scarf in the center of your neck. Then cross the ends in the back and bring them to the front. Loop them over one another or knot them for the look you like.

The same long scarf folded on the bias can be made into a man's tie. Begin by putting the scarf around your neck, points in the front, with the left end shorter than the right. Hold the left end in your left hand. With your right hand wrap the right end over the left two times. Keep the right end in your right hand and put the end through the V. Pull it up through the V, then put it through the loop and pull down. Hold the left end in your left hand and push the knot up with your right hand. You can wear it close to your neck or looser and further down.

Any size square can be tied into a cowboy style. Fold your scarf into a triangle and knot the ends. Move the knotted ends to the back and the triangle to the front.

The square shape can also be folded horizontally and made into an ascot. Fold into an oblong and bring it around the neck. Flip one end over the other and it will be a fluffy ascot. The oblong scarf also makes a good ascot. Bring the scarf around your neck and then loop one end over the other. The ascot can be worn outside your collar or tucked in for a tailored look. It can be worn under sweater collars as well as shirts to bring more color and pattern to your outfit.

The oblong scarf can be used to create the hacking style. Fold the oblong in half. With both ends to one side, bring it around your neck. Take both ends and pull them through the doubled loop. Pull the ends to move the loop up as tight as you like.

To make a full bow, tie an oblong scarf as you would tie a bow. Then pull out the fabric of the bow so that it is as wide and floppy as you like. Wear it in front or to the side.

You can also use two oblongs together. Either lay them flat or twist them together. Then tie them into an ascot, a muffler or a bow. Use two solid colors, a solid and a pattern or even two compatible patterns together.

If you have an oversized square or oblong, wear it over one shoulder for a dressy look. Place it over your shoulder and belt it. Or wear it loose and let it hang softly. The best material is a soft wool or challis which will cling to your dress or top.

Scarves can be used to finish an outfit or soften a look. You may want to keep certain shades near your face because you know they complement your hair or skin or eyes. A scarf is the perfect way to accomplish this. You'll find that you don't always have to wear the prescribed colors in your suits and dresses if you wear scarves in flattering shades. For instance, if your best colors are peach and turquoise, use these for a bow at the neck or an ascot, and choose stronger or darker colors for your clothes. If you prefer jackets and skirts or dresses in neutrals such as navy and gray, don't be afraid to highlight your face with brighter colored neckwear. The right-colored bow will add vitality to your appearance.

Use your scarves to change the mood of your clothes. If you're going out after work, try a large shawl over one shoulder, or a glittery muffler or oversized bow at the neck. These accessories dress up your outfit and help you feel as if you've changed your clothes without really doing so. Wear them during the work day to coordinate your clothes. You can easily wear unmatched skirts and jackets if you tie your outfit together with your neckwear; a simple bow at the neck that coordinates with the color of your skirt will lend an appearance of unity to your outfit. Scarves are an inexpensive tactic to manage your wardrobe and signal your style.

COATS. A coat should be considered as an essential element in your Capsule. More than just a cover-up, it should be good-looking, protect you from the elements, and coordinate with your Capsule. It usually represents a significant investment, and as such, it should work with all of your clothes, functioning as a complementary component of your wardrobe.

Before shopping for outerwear, assess your needs. First of all, determine the weather conditions and the frequency with which you need a coat. If you live in the northeast or midwest, you obviously need a warm coat to wear almost every day during the winter over your working wardrobe. You may also need a second coat for milder, rainy weather, particularly in the spring. If you live in the sunbelt, you may only need a raincoat. However, if you travel to colder climates, you may need a raincoat with a button-out lining.

Consider the style of your clothes; they should definitely be a factor in the style of coat you buy. If you wear soft, knitted clothes, then a soft coat will look best over them. A tailored coat would look stiff and rigid. If you wear mostly suits and crisp dresses, then your coat should have a similar look.

Coordinate your coat with the colors of your Capsule. If you're going to use your coat for both daytime and evening, a dark color may be appropriate. Colors such as black and navy look smart during the day and dressy at night. Generally speaking, brown, beige, tan, wine, red, blue, or green all look fine for work but are less elegant in the evening.

Decide how much money you want to spend. If you need two coats, you may want to invest more in the coat you wear all winter than the one you only need in the spring. But if you're going to use the raincoat for evening as well as during the daytime, you may decide it is worthwhile to invest more money in it. Consider coats that have more than one function. For instance, a black nylon coat can be worn for rain as well as for evening. It can be excellent as a packable travel coat too. A trenchcoat with a button-out lining may be effective for wet weather and for cold weather, but it is usually too casual to wear over dressy evening clothes.

Once you have a clear objective, you can be more specific when you begin to shop. There are three factors to consider when trying on a coat: color, fabric and style. The colors of your Capsule should determine the color of your coat. It is generally most effective to choose the darker color in your Capsule. For instance, if your base colors are black and red, the black will work with all of your clothes and look appropriate if you are going out in the evening. If your base colors are lighter, such as tan and gray, then either one will do, especially since both of these are neutral colors. From a practical standpoint, a darker color is preferable, particularly if you travel. It will not show dirt as easily and can be used in many different situations. If you have more than one Capsule in your wardrobe, try to choose the darkest color that will work with all of them. One word of caution on the colors in your Capsules— if you are considering black or navy as a base color, choose one and not both. Either color is excellent and accessories in those colors will work with other Capsules as well, but black and navy rarely work with each other.

The second factor in selecting a coat is the fabric. For cold weather protection, 100 percent wool, cashmere, alpaca, vicuna or camel's hair is best. They'll keep you warm in the winter, yet because these natural fibers breathe, they can be comfortable even when the weather is slightly warmer. Synthetic fibers such as polyester will not slough off the cold. Layers of natural fibers, such as a cotton coat with a wool lining, also offer good protection. And one of the best types of outerwear for cold or wet weather is a fur-lined coat.

Third, consider the style of the coat. When you're trying on a coat, always wear a jacket or heavy sweater under it. Chances are this is how you'll wear it on cold or rainy days. Although salespeople often suggest that you take off your jacket before trying on a coat, you should not. It may seem more comfortable (especially if you're trying a winter coat on a balmy fall day), but it isn't realistic. In fact, if you aren't wearing a jacket, borrow one from the store.

There are several different styles to look for, and all of them should fit you comfortably and easily. If you have to squeeze yourself into a coat, it isn't right for you. There should be plenty of arm and shoulder room so that you don't feel stiff or look like a toy soldier. The coat should be long enough to cover your longest skirts and dresses. The prettiest coat in the world looks terrible when the hem of your dress is hanging beneath it.

If your clothes lean towards the crisp side, you may prefer a reefer, a chesterfield, a polo, a balmacaan or a trenchcoat style. These are straight cut, menswear looks that go well with suits and tailored dresses. If you wear softer clothes, consider a wrap style or a coat with a full, swinging back or a cape. If you wear many knits, then a cape or knit coat may coordinate best. There are some knit coats that are reversible and give you a completely different look. Typically, cotton, leather or polyurethane are used on the reverse side of the knit.

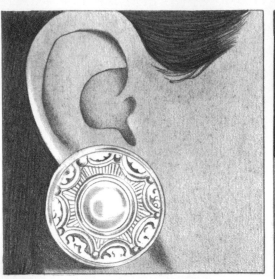
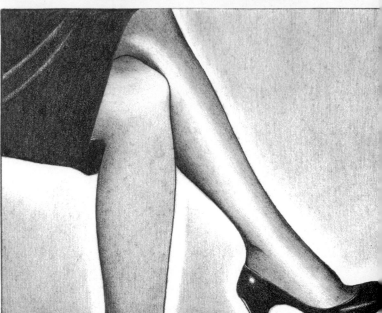
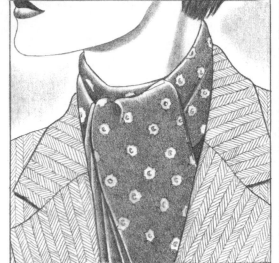
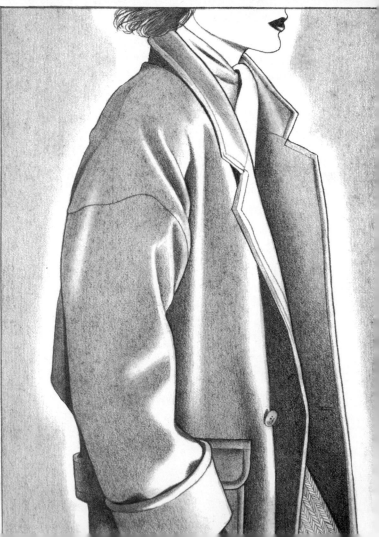
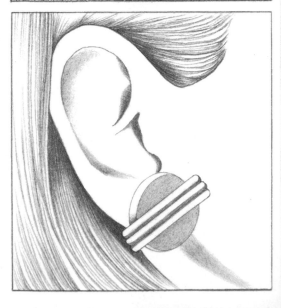

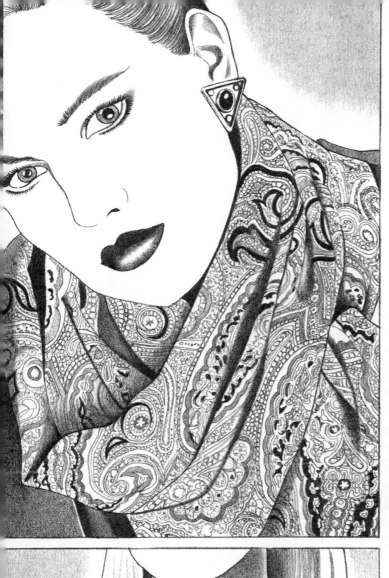
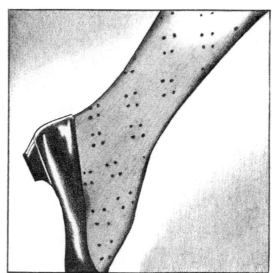
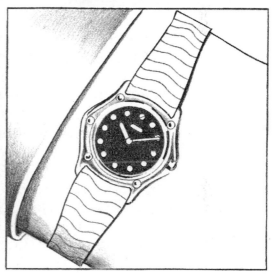
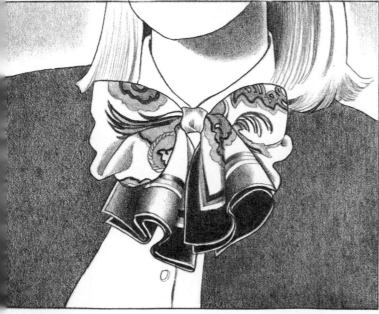
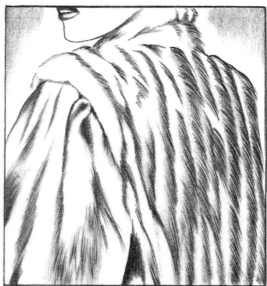

Knits can be excellent for travel too, particularly in reversible styles. If you travel a great deal, or need a raincoat as often as a warmer coat, then consider a trenchcoat with a button-out lining. Many good-looking raincoats are now being made of polyurethane or rubber or even coated plastic. Another alternative, especially suited to travel, is a double coat composed of a lightweight outer shell with a wool or fur coat underneath.

When buying a fur coat, use the same guidelines you would follow for buying a cloth one. The color is very important and should be flattering to your skin, eyes and hair. Try on a variety of furs in different shades to see what is most attractive on you. Shape is also important. You may want a fur coat that is tailored enough to wear to work every day, or decide on a style that is dressier and can be worn more for evenings. If you are buying a fur to wear to work, be sure to try it on over a jacket or bulky sweater, just as you would with a cloth coat.

Fur coats have now become the domain of working women. For many years, women waited for the men in their lives to buy them a fur. But now as more women earn their own money, furs have become a part of the successful working woman's wardrobe. In colder climates, particularly in the northeast and midwest, fur coats are a practical way to deal with extremely cold weather. A well-made, durable fur coat can give you years of return on your investment. Some environmentalists are opposed to furs, and you should be aware of the possibility of offending someone by wearing a fur coat. Furs that are sold in the United States, however, come from animals bred specially for fur-bearing, and usually aren't made from pelts of endangered species.

There are a wide variety of furs to choose from. If you are buying a fur coat, make sure your first one is in a classic style that will look attractive for years to come. Don't invest a lot of money in a trendy fur that may look out of style next year.

Three of the most popular and durable furs are raccoon, beaver and mink. These last for many years and provide both warmth and good looks. Raccoon and beaver are less costly than fine mink, but are not as dressy. Japanese raccoon, called Tanuki, is a reddish color that is more unusual than the typical gray raccoon, but it is not as long-lasting. Beaver is a shorter-haired fur that is heavier than raccoon or mink, and generally less expensive.

Many women consider the most practical fur (from a long-term investment point of view) to be mink. It is durable, warm, and, in a classic cut, it doesn't go out of style. Buying a mink coat can be confusing: They are advertised at prices that range from a few thousand dollars to twenty or thirty thousand dollars. Just as clothing can be inexpensive or very expensive, there is a difference in low-priced and higher-priced minks. The most expensive mink coats are made of female skins. The female skins are smaller than the male skins and it takes more of them to make up a coat. At the same time, they are lighter in weight and so more comfortable to wear. The higher-priced minks are a natural color (no dyes or color added), and the skins have a luster to them. In addition, the style of the coat, the length of it, and the way it is sewn together all contribute to the cost. Coats made of fully let-out skins are the finest; it is far less expensive to use scraps and paws to make coats that are pieced together. The best minks are bred in the United States and sewn together here. Several manufacturers of lower-priced minks are making coats in the Orient and then shipping them back to the U.S. Many of these coats are not up to the quality of American-made furs, so it is important to know where a fur coat has been made.

Other long-haired furs which are popular are fox and lynx. These are more delicate than mink or raccoon, shed more easily, and usually do not last as long. But they are very attractive furs which look and feel luxurious. In more expensive furs, lynx and sable are becoming even more desirable than they were in the past. Both of these are extremely durable, classic furs which can last for many, many years. One reason that sable is so expensive is that the best sables are bred only in the Soviet Union. Auctions for sable are held twice a year there, prices are in dollars only, and fur traders from all over the world come to bid on them.

When you are buying a fur coat, shop around, ask questions, and look for seasonal sales. You'll probably see an enormous differential in the price of fur coats, so be prepared to find out what the reasons are. Usually, you get what you pay for. High-quality furs that are well-made do cost more, but they look better, last longer, and even retain a higher resale value. As with anything else you buy, you should have confidence in the company you buy your fur from, and feel secure that you can rely on them should you need your coat altered or repaired.

There is no question that a fur coat makes a strong statement about its wearer. Wearing a fur, like mink, fisher or sable, immediately implies money and suggests that you are a successful woman. Lighter-colored furs, such as fox and lynx, may be too flamboyant for most

Corporate or Communicator profiles. Keep in mind that darker furs such as mink may fit in better with a traditional business look. Some women find that wearing a fur coat to the boardroom or high-powered meetings, and on social occasions with colleagues, establishes their authority and rank. At the same time, wearing a fur when you want to build a rapport with someone who cannot afford fur may only bring about resentment. Be discreet.

Nancy Reynolds (partner in her own high-powered lobbying firm) says she won't wear a fur coat when lobbying on Capitol Hill. But Patti Mancini (vice president of Rockwell International) also visits Congress and isn't afraid to wear a fur as she feels it reinforces her company's strong financial position.

As Leonard Hankin of Maximillian Furs told me, "If a young woman is going for a job interview at a law firm, wearing a fur coat may stop her from getting past the first secretary." Once she has that job, however, her fur coat may help her image with clients as a successful attorney.

How Sharp Is Your Shopping?

Take this quiz to see how sharp your shopping strategy is.

1. When you go into a store do you:

a) Feel dizzy and run out ☐
b) Feel so confused you can't get past cosmetics ☐
c) Head directly for the department you want ☐

2. In the dressing room do you:

a) Feel depressed when you see yourself in the mirror ☐
b) Take in so much you don't know where to begin ☐
c) Feel like they never make clothes for you ☐
d) Love what you try on; buy just what you need ☐

3. When you go shopping do you:

a) Know you need a whole new wardrobe ☐
b) Know you need some things but aren't sure what ☐
c) Think you may need a skirt but don't know what color ☐
d) Know you need a white blouse ☐

4. When you buy a jacket, does it:

a) Look like all the jackets you already own ☐
b) Look like it belongs in someone else's closet ☐
c) Go with only one skirt you own ☐
d) Coordinate with most of your wardrobe ☐

5. When you buy something on sale:

a) It's usually a drastic mistake ☐
b) You may be able to wear it to a costume party ☐
c) It may be something you can use ☐
d) It is exactly what you needed ☐

6. When you buy a blouse it is:

a) The wrong color; you didn't remember the color of your skirt ☐
b) The right color but the style doesn't go with your skirt ☐
c) Pretty, but it doesn't go with anything you own ☐
d) The right blouse to go with most of your clothes ☐

7. When you need a blouse do you:

a) Never find a blouse you like ☐
b) Buy a blouse, a dress and a sweater ☐
c) Buy a new lipstick ☐
d) Buy the blouse ☐

8. When you are shopping for clothes do you:

a) Look for a smaller size; you'll lose weight ☐
b) Wish you had a different job ☐
c) Wish you could throw out all your clothes ☐
d) Find some nice things and try them on ☐

9. Before you shop for a new season:

a) You have no idea of what's in fashion ☐
b) You have no idea of what's in your closet ☐
c) You think you need some new shoes ☐
d) You read magazines, look at store displays ☐

10. Do you shop:

a) When it's so crowded you can never get any help ☐
b) On a lunch hour when you hardly have time ☐
c) After work when you're tired ☐
d) When you have a day off and plenty of time ☐

Score 1 point for each "a"; 3 points for each "b"; 5 points for each "c"; 7 points for each "d". EVALUATION: *10–25—Reread this book; 26–50—Rethink your wardrobe, start building Capsules; 51–65—Organize your closet and make a buying plan; 56–70—Great!*

CHAPTER XI

Strategies for Shopping

Nearly every woman has some insecurities about shopping. Anxieties may take various forms—from feeling dizzy at the sight of racks of clothing to never going near a store. Some of the anxiety has to do with making choices in clothing; some with spending money; some with facing your figure; some with your self-image.

When you buy clothes, you are deciding how you want to present yourself to the world. Corporations spend millions of dollars researching how to package their products. What you wear makes a major statement about *your* package—you. Having to choose which of all the available items in the various stores are the ones that depict you best is a decision of great consequence. If you're going to be perceived as a competent, promotable career woman, you have to present the right picture. If you want to have credibility with clients or show your assertiveness, you've got to dress the part.

Making those decisions while shopping on a lunch hour and your eye is on the clock is not being fair to yourself. For many working women, shopping is a chore, a necessary eventuality squeezed into an already overloaded agenda. A generation ago, women shopped to socialize, to entertain themselves and even to gratify themselves. Ironically, they could spend the time because they didn't have careers. But for today's women, shopping is done on a rushed lunch hour or on a busy weekend. Your time is limited, your budget may be tight, and yet your wardrobe is essential to your success.

After spending hundreds of dollars and as many hours, you may find you have a closet full of clothes and nothing to wear. You can solve this problem by developing a shopping strategy. Let's look at some difficulties faced by real women and come up with a program for solving their problems.

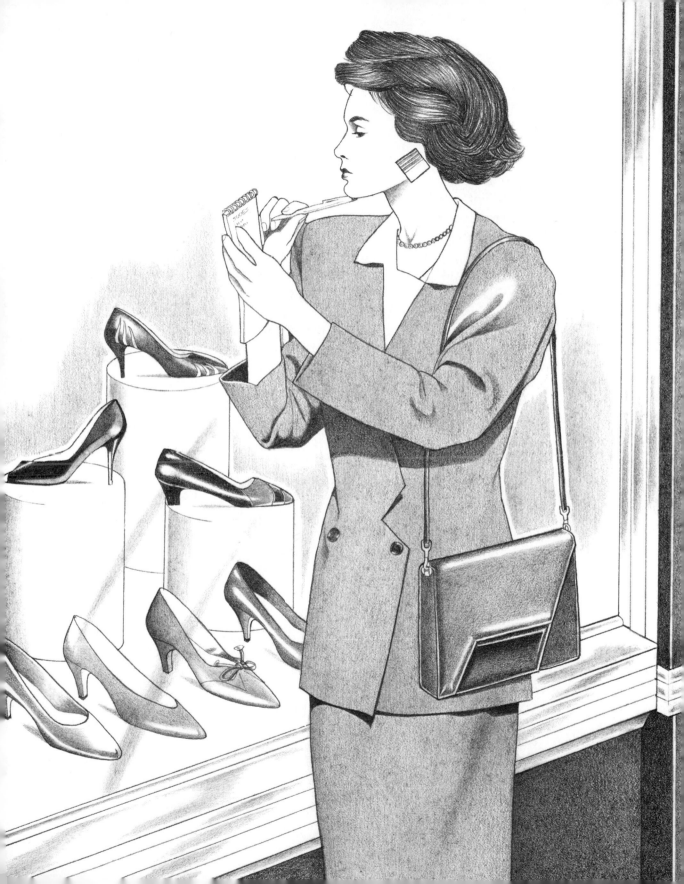

PROBLEM: "I never know what to buy. If I see something I like, I don't know if it will go with what I have at home. I usually wind up with the wrong thing."

SOLUTION: Start with a plan. When professional store buyers begin a new season, they work out a plan of what clothes they have on hand in their department, what did well last year, and what they think they'll need this year. They write down how much money they have to spend, which categories they're going to spend it in, and how they'll divide their dollars among jackets, skirts, blouses, shoes, etc.

You can do the same thing. Be organized and make a buying plan. This is a business move, as strategic to your career as your planning guide or your goals. When you buy clothing, you're making an investment even though it may not seem that way. But add up your clothing bill for a few years; you may find it is as much as you have in your savings account or invested in the stock market.

Begin with what is already in your closet. Be realistic. When merchandise doesn't sell, the buyers take markdowns to get it out of their stock. That way it doesn't tie up their capital or valuable floor space. Be honest with yourself. If you have clothes that you haven't worn in the last three years, cut your losses and get them out of your closet. Then you'll feel free to make new purchases. Take the clothes you don't wear and put them aside. If you don't like the colors, feel they don't flatter you, feel uncomfortable when you wear them, know they're out of style, or realize they're simply worn out, then get rid of them. Be generous. You'll make someone else happy and you'll feel better too. Donate the clothes you don't wear to a charity, sell them in a resale shop, or give them to someone you know. Acknowledge your mistakes. Once you do, you'll no longer feel guilty every time you open your closet door and face those expensive errors. Grit your teeth, get them out, and get on with the business of managing your wardrobe.

List the clothes you wear by color and components, writing down skirts, jackets, blouses, sweaters and dresses. If you have a Capsule or even the beginning of one, list the pieces in that Capsule by color. Be aware of the kinds of clothes that are successful for you: the fabrics, colors and styles you like.

Now make a separate list of the items you need. Think about what kinds of pieces will complete your Capsule. Check your shoes and your handbags. Make sure they go with the clothes in your Capsule. Be specific about your needs. If you go shopping because you "need something," but aren't sure what that something is, you can waste precious hours of time and hard earned dollars in frustration. We all have a tendency to pick up an item here and there, attracted by its color or fabric, encouraged because it is very much in style (and looks perfect on someone else), only to discover later that it goes with absolutely nothing we own. Restrain yourself, or at least limit these impulses to small, inexpensive acccssories. They, at least, can help you update your clothes without the considerable expensc of a new wardrobe. A new scarf, new earrings, or new necklace can act as an emotional pick-me-up and do the same for your Capsule.

When you go shopping, wear or bring along at least one outfit from your Capsule. If you are working with a pattern, this is particularly important. You may have a skirt or jacket in a multicolored pattern that includes several colors such as red, blue, yellow and green. You'll find that when you put a red top with it, it looks one way, but looks very different with a green top. Each color brings out different shades in the pattern; when you combine colors, they change. It is often difficult to recall the exact cast or undertones of colors. You may visualize what you have at home as very different from what it actually is. When you have something with you, such as a skirt, a jacket or a dress, it is much easier to blend it, contrast it, or combine it with other pieces. When professional fashion people, like designers, coordinators and stylists, put outfits together they keep the clothes in front of them. They don't leave things up to their memories and you shouldn't either.

PROBLEM: "Sometimes I buy something in a store, then later see my friend wearing something I like better."

SOLUTION: At the start of the season, professional buyers go on a scouting expedition. They shop the whole market to see what their resources are offering, who has the best styles, the best fabrics and the best prices.

Do likewise. At the beginning of the season, when most of the merchandise is in stock, scout the stores in your area to see what they are offering. Even if they carry the same manufacturers, they'll have different items from those lines. Take your buying plan so you know what you need. But don't buy. Just look. Then you can decide who has the best selection to fill your needs. When you are ready to spend your money, you'll know what your options are.

PROBLEM: "When I do find something I like, I can never afford it."

SOLUTION: Make a budget. Professional buyers know exactly how much they have to spend and which categories they will spend it on. Once in a while, if they see something special, they may exceed their budget, but only if they know it will pay off in dividends.

Figure out what items you need and then decide how much to spend in each area. Give yourself some leeway. You may find a skirt that is $30 more than you wanted to spend but is absolutely perfect with your whole Capsule. On the other hand, you may be able to buy your shoes on sale, or do without an item which is not as essential.

Think in terms of a "Lifetime Wearings Ratio." If an item is expensive but you will wear it often, over a long period of time, it is a worthwhile investment. Basics, such as well-made blouses, fall into this category. An item that's cheap, and that you'll only wear once, may not be worth the money. Something that's expensive, such as an evening gown that you will wear only two or three times over a period of years, may also be a poor investment. Smart shoppers spend more on clothes they wear frequently and can use for a long time than on items they'll rarely wear.

Look for quality. It may be true that the clothes that appeal to you *are* over your budget. Rethink your buying plan and buy fewer but better components. A well-made jacket will look elegant and can last for years. It may cost more than a moderate-priced jacket, but you'll be getting more than a dollar for dollar return. Remember too, amortize your investment. If you are spending more but look better and can get more years of wear, then it is a better value.

Don't get hung up on having lots of clothes. You can make your clothes look very different if you have interchangeable pieces. Accessories can also make a big difference in an outfit. One good skirt can look different every day of the week if you change the tops and the accessories. Concentrate on quality, not quantity.

Buy clothes that can be returned. Unless you are absolutely, positively sure of something, don't risk not being able to bring it back.

Most department stores will take things back even if you bought them on sale, if you return them within a reasonable period of time. If you aren't sure of store policy, ask the salesperson. Be cautious shopping in discount stores or small specialty stores where purchases are final. However, if you know exactly what you want—style, size and color—then discounters can save you money. They are best for labeled merchandise with which you're already familiar. Shop the department stores first so you'll know what's available; then go to the discount outlets. Or wait for sales; markdowns in department stores have become so prevalent that you can frequently find a good buy there.

PROBLEM: "The stores present such a confusing picture. Everything looks the same. There may be five floors filled with blouses; it's hard to know where to begin. There are racks and racks of clothes."

SOLUTION: Scout the store. Before going in, take a minute and look at the windows for new ideas. Merchants use their windows and mannequins as an advertising and educational vehicle. The more their customers see and know, the more likely they are to buy. This is where buyers put their newest merchandise, styling it in the most fashionable way. Each mannequin may tell more than one story. The display may show color or style trends, feature new fashion designers, or emphasize new accessories. Take advantage of this information so that you learn how to make the clothes you already own look new. If you like the new looks, think about what you already have and how you can update your wardrobe.

Once inside the store, look around. Become familiar with the different departments so you know what type of merchandise is offered in each. If you are very interested in new ideas or what's in fashion, go to the designer departments. Even if you can't afford the clothes, touch them and try them on to see what makes them special. This will help you when you go to the more moderate departments. You'll know what is in fashion, which styles and colors look new and which look old, and what is well-made. Each season designers put together new color combinations, new proportions and new fabric mixtures and it's important to be able to spot them.

Very often people ask me if there are rules for what fabrics go together. I tell them to look at the trends for the season because the very nature of fashion is change. One year a shiny charmeuse blouse looks great with a gabardine skirt. The next year a matte finish looks much better. Proportions change the same way. One season a long jacket looks best with a long full skirt. The next year it looks fresh and new when the skirt is short and straight. That doesn't mean that each season you must go out and buy new clothes. It does mean that each season you should reevaluate what is in your closet, rethink what goes together, and experiment with colors, proportions and textures.

PROBLEM: "I never know what to buy. Fashion is so confusing. I'm not the trendy type, but I do want to be in style. I'm always a year behind. Then too, if you buy something basic it's boring, but if it's fashionable, the next season it goes out of style."

SOLUTION: Let your eye adjust to new ideas. Read the fashion magazines such as *Vogue, Harper's Bazaar* and *Glamour*. You'll get a feeling for the direction of fashion. Also read career women's magazines such as *Working Woman, Ms.* and *Savvy* for more conservative career dressing.

As you shop the stores, look for ways to adapt the fashion information to your working and leisure wardrobes. Only by seeing new trends will you get used to them. If the current fashion is baggy pants, and the newest ones are skinny, it will take a while to get accustomed to the narrow look. But after seeing them over and over, they begin to look right. Eventually the baggy pants look tired and out of style. Fashion professionals see looks repeated again and again in runway shows. A designer may show dozens of variations on a theme to get his or her point across. For instance, one season Giorgio Armani may have a new collar for his jackets. He'll show it on brown jackets, black jackets, blue jackets and gray jackets. One after another, mannequins walk down the runway wearing different jackets but all with that same collar. It doesn't take long before buyers and editors get the message. You can learn by observing what is in the stores and what the trendsetters are wearing.

Some cities are more attuned to fashion than others, and it is easier to see what the new styles are. Take a walk on Madison Avenue, Columbus Avenue or West Broadway and you will quickly learn what the latest trends are for the people who frequent those areas of New York. The same applies to Rodeo Drive in Beverly Hills or North Michigan Avenue in Chicago. You can get dozens of ideas for smart dressing just by standing in one place for a while. Very often, Bill Cunningham, the fashion photographer for the *New York Times,* stands at the corner of 57th Street and Fifth Avenue, his camera ready to catch the latest looks. In other cities, where the trends are not so visible, use the designer departments of fashion stores as a source of information. Here again the fashion magazines can be a big help. This doesn't mean that you must dress "trendy," but even the Corporate woman can use some of these ideas to update her clothes. You may adapt new proportions, buy a new color, change to a flatter heel, or even try a new way of tying a scarf.

PROBLEM: "They never have the clothes I like in my size."

SOLUTION: Going shopping means facing your figure. We all have lumps and bumps, and although your friends can mysteriously get away with them, your own always seem to be in the wrong places. Trying on new clothes brings your figure faults into focus and the reality is often painful and depressing.

Forget about size tags and concentrate on the clothes. Be willing to try different sizes. Every manufacturer cuts his clothes with a different pattern. You may wear a size fourteen from one firm and a size twelve from another. When styles change, the sizes change too. One lawyer who usually wears a size fourteen told me a saleswoman found a wonderful skirt for her in a size ten. She never would have found the skirt for herself because she never would have looked at the clothes marked size ten. But the saleswoman knew how fully that skirt was cut.

More expensive clothes are usually cut fuller than less expensive ones, so you may wear one or two sizes less in higher-priced garments. One reason clothes go on sale is that they may be cut differently from the size marked on them. Look at everything—especially when clothes are on sale. They may be much larger or much smaller than what they are marked. If you like a style but aren't sure it will fit, try it on.

Remember that clothes can be altered. Few women can immediately wear the clothes they buy. Most of us need some alterations, whether it's hems, sleeves, waistlines or hips. There is nothing wrong with alterations. Men almost always require some adjustments on their clothes. After all, manufacturers make clothes to fit thousands of people, and we are, fortunately, not all built exactly the same.

Find a good seamstress. If you don't know one, ask well-dressed women you meet for the names of their seamstresses. Sooner or later you'll find someone who is good. She not only will alter your clothes, but she may be able to reproduce your favorite styles from other colors and fabrics.

Shop early in the season. If you wait until the last minute, you won't find the selection that the stores have when the merchandise first arrives. Especially if you are a very small or very large size, try not to wait too long. When department store buyers take one dozen of a particular style, they usually buy only one piece of the smallest size and one piece of the largest size. No wonder those sizes sell quickly!

Keep an eye out for what you need. If you know that you can use a long black skirt for evening and you see one that's well-priced and fits, buy it, even if you have no special evenings planned. You won't be sorry. The same thing applies for classic skirts, well-made cotton or silk blouses, simple dresses and basic shoes, belts, and handbags. Certain clothes and accessories are staples in your wardrobe. If you don't wear them right now, chances are you'll wear them next week or next month and often after that. These basics will be amortized over a period of years.

PROBLEM: "Finding the right salesperson is like playing hide and seek. All too often stores that say they offer service simply don't. The lack of good salespeople is appalling. When I do find someone to help me, it often seems that they know less than I do. And if they do show me clothes, they look as if they're for three other people. The salespeople don't take the time or the interest to look at me and understand my needs."

SOLUTION: Look for a saleswoman who you think is well-dressed. That is one indication that she cares about the clothes she sells. Chances are she can help you find clothes that appeal to you. Tell her what you need and what you already have. This will help her to help you. Personal shoppers or fashion consultants go so far as to make a file for their customers, listing all their clothes, what they buy, and even where they wear them. The more a saleswoman knows about you, the more she can help you find the right styles. If you go out often after work, tell her. If your clothes are strictly for the office, let her know. Don't be afraid to say how much you want to spend. Otherwise she may be heading in the wrong direction, picking clothes that are out of your reach. Ask her how to put the clothes together. If she is professional and understands the clothes she is selling, she will be able to show you how to get more than one outfit from what you are buying. Ask her for other pieces to put with the new clothes. She may be able to pull together four or five components that will build into an effective Capsule.

When you find salespeople you like, build a relationship with them. Let them know you want to give them your business. In return tell them to call you when merchandise is going on sale and when new clothes come in. Ask them to put aside clothes for you that they think you might like. Many women are learning to rely on one or two stores where they have a favorite salesperson. If that person knows what you like and what you can afford, he or she can save you an enormous amount of time and money. Since salespeople are in the store and are familiar with the merchandise, they are much more aware of what is available than you can be. They know how clothes fit, what other styles can be coordinated with them, and how to accessorize them.

Many stores around the country are now offering executive shopping services for working women. Macy's in New York, Kaufmann's in Pittsburgh, Sanger-Harris in Dallas, the Emporium in San Francisco, Carson Pirie Scott in Chicago, Higbee's in Cleveland, Dayton-Hudson in Detroit, and Garfinckel's in Washington are just a few examples. Call the major stores in your city and ask what services they offer. These services are generally free. Sometimes stores have minimum purchase requirements, but usually they do not. Since the people who work in these areas are trained to dress career women, they can be very helpful. They may also have the freedom to go around the entire store, selecting merchandise from many different departments. They know what clothes and accessories are in stock, and they know how to make them work for you.

Or you may choose to shop in smaller specialty stores that specialize in clothes for career women. These stores are cropping up all over the country and can be very helpful in selecting appropriate clothes. But be sure the clothes they sell are right for you. Don't get bogged down by boring suits and bow ties.

PROBLEM: "Going shopping is so frustrating that I come home depressed and hating myself. The entire experience makes me exhausted. I feel as though there's something wrong with me. It seems as if nothing fits, nothing looks good on me, and nothing is ever available in my size. In desperation I buy something, anything, and I take it home and find it goes with nothing else I own. It sits in my closet and I never wear it."

SOLUTION: Try to shop at off hours. Unfortunately most women only have free time on their lunch hour or on a Saturday or Sunday, so everyone is trying to shop at the same time. If you can reschedule your lunch hour and take it earlier or later in the day, or shop in the evening instead of on the weekend, you may find that the stores are not so crowded. Most women shop toward the week's end. If you shop at the beginning of the week, you may find that the salespeople have more time to help you and the dressing rooms are not so busy.

Don't shop when you are tired. Buying clothes takes a toll on energy and emotions, so try to go shopping when you are feeling fresh. If you are dragging yourself about, you won't want to try things on and you won't have the patience to persevere. Buying the right clothes can sometimes mean trying on dozens of things. It can be emotionally draining to stare at yourself in the mirror and feel as if nothing is made for you. If you are tired you may want to give up. For some women shopping is an energizer, but if it gets you down, don't go if you're feeling depressed already. Better to wait for another time.

Look for a large dressing room with a three way mirror and good lighting. This is easier to say than to find but at least try for one. If you are shopping in an expensive department, insist on it. If the lighting in the dressing room is not good, take the clothes to a window or go out on the selling floor to see the colors better.

Give yourself enough time. If you don't have much time to spend on shopping, you'll tend to buy the first thing that fits. When you get it home, it will more than likely turn out to be the same thing you already have—or something totally wrong for you.

PROBLEM: "A lot of times I buy things and then they go on sale a few weeks later."

SOLUTION: Ask about sales. Very often the saleswoman knows when the merchandise is going to be marked down. It may be that the clothes you like will be going on sale in a week. She may even be able to hold them for you until then or at least call you when the sale starts. Always check the sale racks. There are two types of clothing that usually get marked down. One of these is the fashion forward merchandise that most customers are not ready to wear. Stores bring in these clothes so that their high-fashion customers can buy them and the more conservative customers will see the new trends. The other type of clothes that frequently gets marked down are basic styles that the store may have overbought. This is a good place to find classic blouses, skirts or pants that won't go out of style. Particularly if you like to buy high-quality clothes and can't afford your preferences at regular prices, watch the sale racks for good buys.

Don't be afraid of expensive stores. Some stores take bigger markdowns than others. Watch the sales in your area and see which stores offer the best buys. Many women who don't buy at retail prices tell me that they get real bargains at better stores such as Neiman-Marcus, Lord & Taylor and Saks Fifth Avenue when those stores run sales.

PROBLEM: "The stores are always advertising sales but half the time the merchandise looks like junk."

SOLUTION: Know when a sale is a sale. Stores have three kinds of sales. One is a legitimate markdown, taken on regular-priced merchandise that customers did not buy. Retailers can only afford to have this merchandise sitting in their stores for so long. After a while they must get their money out of it so that they can buy new goods. The longer they wait the more stale, worn and handled the clothes get, the less likely people are to purchase them, and the greater the markdowns.

The second type of sale is a manufacturer's closeout. These clothes are brought in at regular price with the intention to mark them down after a limited period. Because of Federal Trade Commission laws, merchandise can only be advertised as sale goods if it has been on the selling floor for a specific period of time at a higher price. A typical advertisement for this type of sale will say, "Special purchase. Fifty percent off Famous-Maker clothes. Regularly priced at $100. Now only $50." These sales often come about because the manufacturer, optimistic that certain styles will be in demand that season, has cut more garments than he has been able to sell. Towards the end of the season, when he sees that there are no more orders coming in for these styles, he may approach a store and ask if they are interested in these clothes at a special price. Since this usually happens at the end of the season, you may find that the wearing time is not as long as if you had bought it a few months earlier. It is only a good buy if you can amortize your purchase. If you only get to wear your clothes a few times before you must put them away until the next year, you have tied up your money. If, however, you can still get a lot of wear out of your new clothes for this season, or know you will be depending on them heavily next season, then you have invested wisely.

A third type of sale is a special purchase. Here the buyer may have garments made especially for the store. Because she orders in large enough quantities, the manufacturer may give the store a special price. When this happens you may get a good buy. The price may also be cheaper than similar merchandise because the quality of the fabric is slightly lower than usual, or the styles are less detailed, or the cut is skimpier. Be aware of these variables before you buy.

PROBLEM: "I don't mind shopping for fashion but the basics bore me."

SOLUTION: Use mail order catalogues for your basics. Every good store has them and they usually feature the classic styles that they know will sell. This is a good way to buy silk shirts, cotton blouses, sweaters, and intimate apparel. If you see a style you like, buy it in more than one color. Don't be afraid of repeating it. It looks different in each color.

PROBLEM: "My friends wear some clothes that look so good on them. I can never find styles that are right for me."

SOLUTION: Learn the labels that are right for your figure. Most manufacturers are consistent in their sizes and cut. Some specialize in clothes for a fuller figure, others for a slighter build. For example, Halston makes clothes for women who have full figures. His skirts and pants often have elasticized waists, his jackets often have full backs, and his dress styles are very often loose or straight with little or no waistline. Even his evening clothes are often loose-fitting caftans, styled for women with fuller figures such as Elizabeth Taylor or Liza Minelli. On the other hand, Albert Nipon dresses are cut for a smaller woman. Pearl Nipon, the designer for the firm, is short and small boned. She designs clothes that would suit her. The firm also makes extra small sizes like twos and fours which are hard to find. In addition, many firms are now making petite collections for women who are 5′4″ and under.

Since so many women are moving back and forth between career profiles, be aware that the clothes you buy need not be locked into one look. A navy suit need not be typecast forever as a Corporate component. Nevertheless, there are certain well-known names which can be identified with certain classifications, and others which fall between two profiles. Following are some of the labels to look for when you go shopping, whether in person or by mail or phone. Obviously, new designers and manufacturers are always coming on the market. But the list below should be helpful as a guideline to each profile. When you are in the stores, look for these labels and become familiar with their style and cut. If you know that certain manufacturers make clothes for your style and figure, you can cut your shopping time in half.

CORPORATE PROFILE

Adolfo	Cricketeer	John Henry
Aquascutum	David Hayes	Kasper
Arthur Chapnik	Ernst Strauss	Louis Feraud
Betty Hanson	Evan Picone	St. John
Castleberry	Harvé Benard	Saint Laurie
Chaus	Jaeger	Spitalnick
Chanel	J. G. Hook	Yves Saint Laurent

COMMUNICATOR PROFILE

Adolfo	David Hayes	Liz Claiborne
Anne Klein	Ellen Tracy	Louis Feraud
Anne Klein II	Escada	Missoni
Betty Hanson	Evan Picone	Perry Ellis
Bill Blass	Giorgio Armani	Ralph Lauren
Blassport	Gloria Sachs	St. Gillian
Calvin Klein	Jaeger	St. John
Chanel	J. G. Hook	Tahari
Christian Dior	Jones New York	Yves Saint Laurent

CREATIVE PROFILE

Anne Klein	Claude Montana	Krizia
Anne Klein II	Geoffrey Beene	Missoni
Bill Blass	Giorgio Armani	Oscar de la Renta
Calvin Klein	Gloria Sachs	Ralph Lauren
Chanel	Kamali	Yves Saint Laurent

Do You Travel Light?

Take this quiz to see if you are ready for your next trip.

1. When you go away do you:

a) Pack so much you could stay away forever ☐

b) Look as if you could stay away about a month ☐

c) Pack lightly but forget a lot of things ☐

d) Pack lightly and have everything you need ☐

2. When you pack do you:

a) Forget your tooth brush, curlers, and cosmetics ☐

b) Take everything in your medicine cabinet ☐

c) Usually forget a few things ☐

d) Have your necessities pre-packed ☐

3. When you unpack is everything:

a) Upside down and hopelessly wrinkled ☐

b) Pretty wrinkled ☐

c) Not bad except for a few wrinkled things ☐

d) Neat and orderly ☐

4. When you reached your destination did you:

a) Find that one of your bags burst—it was overstuffed ☐

b) Lose your luggage— three people thought it looked like theirs ☐

c) Have a hard time carrying all your bags ☐

d) Have your luggage and grab the first taxi ☐

5. When you arrived at your meeting did you feel:

a) Dressed all wrong for the city ☐

b) Like hiding because your clothes were so wrinkled ☐

c) Inappropriate for that meeting ☐

d) You looked as if you belonged there ☐

6. At the meeting did people think you were:

a) A lower ranking member of the firm than you are ☐

b) The boss's girlfriend ☐

c) Someone new in the company ☐

d) The future head of the firm ☐

7. On your trip did you:

a) Bring winter clothes and it was hot and humid ☐

b) Count on a hair-dresser but they were closed ☐

c) Wish you had brought comfortable clothes for the weekend ☐

d) Have just the right outfit for a last minute dinner date ☐

8. When you got dressed in the morning:

a) None of your clothes went together ☐

b) Your clothes went together but you forgot the right shoes ☐

c) You had one decent outfit ☐

d) You had several choices ☐

9. On your last trip your suitcase was:

a) So heavy you almost broke your back ☐

b) So heavy you had to wheel it ☐

c) Hard to carry with all your other bags ☐

d) Light enough to carry easily ☐

Score 1 point for each "a"; 3 points for each "b"; 5 points for each "c"; 7 points for each "d". EVALUATION: *9 points— Read this book again; 10–27 points—Read the travel chapter carefully; 28–45—You can plan better with a little effort; 46–63—You win frequent flier points.*

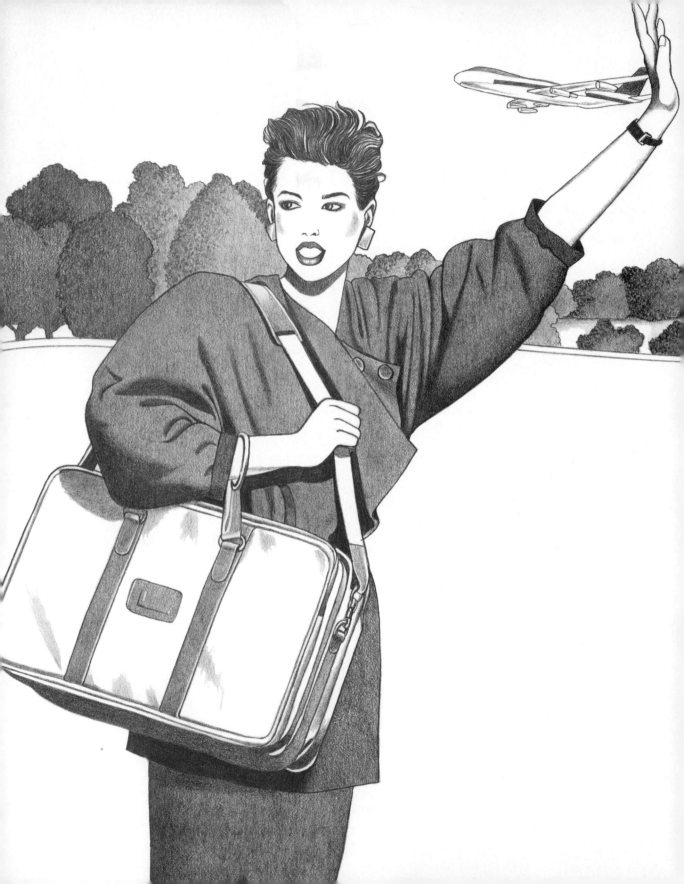

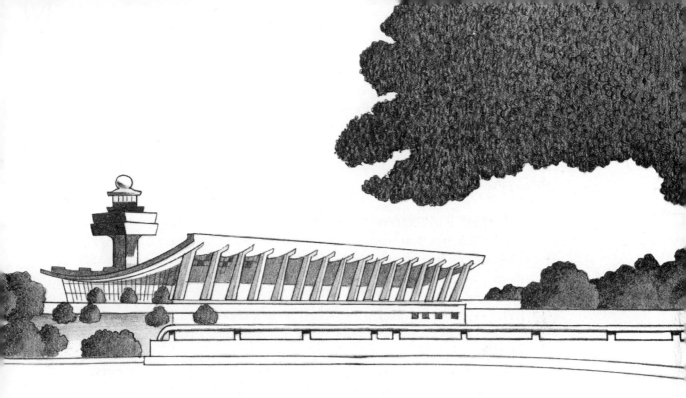

CHAPTER XII

Business Travel

On-the-job traveling has become part of the routine of many work-ing women, not only quick trips to nearby towns, but also over-nights in distant cities or longer stays halfway around the world. Travel can be exciting, adventurous and a growth opportunity if you approach it in an organized way. It can be intimidating and exhaust-ing if you don't.

Before you begin a business trip, find out as much as you can about the city you'll be visiting. Get an idea of the weather and how the natives dress. Ask friends and colleagues what they know about it; if they are familiar with the city, find out their favorite restaurants, shop-ping spots and the best hotels. Learn the names of the local museums, sightseeing musts, special theaters and cultural events.

The most successful trips are those where you feel comfortable. Having everything you need with you makes travel easier and more relaxed. In preparation for your trip, be sure to have a checklist of what you will need. The list that follows is a compilation of the "musts" of many women I've talked to, women who travel frequently as part of their jobs.

- Keep a plastic-lined, multicompartment cosmetic bag always packed with your needs. That way you won't forget necessities at the last minute.
- Use plastic containers with screwtight tops. When you get back home, refill them. Even a spur of the moment trip won't catch you off-guard.
- Keep a few luxuries packed in your cosmetics bag—packages of bubble bath, good soaps, your favorite shampoo and conditioner.
- Use non-spillable items whenever possible—pre-soaked packets of nail polish remover, hairsprays with sealable tops.
- Have a comfortable, lightweight robe for travel. You will want it for room service, for relaxing in after a long day's work, and if the hotel has a swimming pool, you can wear it going from your room to the pool. Take soft, packable slippers; they're much better than walking barefoot in your room.
- Buy luggage you are proud to be seen with. Why feel ashamed of your suitcases when you are met at an airport or checking into a hotel?
- Keep luggage tags on your bags. You may be able to recognize your suitcase, but the next person may not.
- Keep a hand steamer in your suitcase. Many women don't like to travel with silk blouses, silk dresses, wool suits or fancy evening clothes because they are afraid of wrinkles acquired in packing. A hand steamer, unlike an iron, requires only an outlet to plug it into and a little water.
- Take along a good book. It may help you fall asleep at night and it's a good companion if you're lonely. Don't wait until you get there to buy a book; the book selection in airports and hotels can be disappointing at best.
- Always carry your necessities with you. Even if you are checking your luggage, hold onto your cosmetics bag. In the event that your luggage is lost, you will still be able to face the world the next morning.
- Get a hairstyle you can manage yourself; take what you need to keep it looking good. If your hairstyle requires setting your hair, have a small set of electric rollers and/or a blow dryer.
- Use a lingerie bag for your intimate apparel. You can pack your underwear

and nightgowns neatly without getting them squashed, then hang the bag up in your hotel room closet.

- Keep a sachet or potpourri in your suitcase and your clothes will smell fresh.
- Use a jewelry roll for packing earrings, necklaces and bracelets. It will protect them and make it easier to find what you need.
- Use soft, fabric shoe bags to pack your shoes. They will keep your shoes from getting scratched and your clothes from getting dirty.
- Use the following list of travel "musts" as a guideline for packing necessities:

> Skin cleanser
> Skin toner
> Moisturizer
> Facial mask
> Foundation
> Cosmetics
> Nail polish remover pads
> Nail polish and top coat
> Emery board
> Manicure scissors
> Hand cream
> Tweezers
> Toothbrush
> Toothpaste
> Dental floss or travel WaterPik
> Deodorant
> Favorite soap
> Bubble bath
> Sewing kit
> Cotton balls
> Medication/vitamins
> Perfume

Before you pack your clothes, check the weather forecasts for the cities you'll be visiting. You can call the local weather service, or read the weather information in national newspapers.

Next, make a list, by date and time, of the places you're going and the people you'll be with. Include all meetings, meals and social occasions. This will give you a clearer picture of exactly what clothes you need. Obviously, if you are visiting several different cities, you can wear the same clothes more than once. If you are going to be in one place for a long time, take extra accessories to change the look of your clothes.

Once these essentials are in order, you can focus on your clothes. Think in terms of a Travel Capsule, i.e. a multi-function wardrobe that will take you from work to leisure activities with a minimal number of components. Like your other Capsules, this one should be based on two colors and interchangeable pieces. The cardinal rule for a Travel Capsule is to include pieces that can be worn at least three different ways. For instance, pack a skirt that goes with three different tops, a blouse that works with all of your skirts and pants, and a coat that goes over everything. By using two colors, you can limit the number of shoes and handbags you take with you. Some people seem to leave nothing at home when they travel. This was wonderful in the days of ocean liners, steamer trunks and servants, but today traveling light is essential. The Travel Capsule helps keep your suitcase light enough to carry yourself if necessary.

Begin with your most important pieces, the clothes that you need for work. When you are traveling, your audience is an important consideration in the way you dress. If you're dealing with people you've not met before, try to find out as much about them as you can. Consider too what your role will be—whether you should look authoritative, affable or creative.

If you are a Corporate woman, your Travel Capsule should include at least one matching suit look. If your trip is for one or two days, try to limit yourself to one jacket and skirt. However, if you plan to be away two or more days, with meetings involving the same people, include a second jacket and skirt. Even if your trip is for a week, you can use the two jackets and two skirts as matched suits and as coordinated suits, so that they may be all you need.

The Communicator may not need a matched suit, depending on the purpose of your trip. If you are giving a speech to a Corporate group such as a financial or legal organization where the stress is on power, wear a matched suit. If you are on a sales trip, consider a less rigid look with a coordinated jacket and skirt.

The Creative woman who is going to be away overnight should include an extra top to change her look. If you're going to be with a Corporate group, take a jacket to give you a look of authority.

Any woman going away overnight should take at least one extra blouse. For trips up to a week, plan on one blouse for every day you are away. Even for trips that last longer, four or five blouses will give you sufficient opportunity for changes, and you'll feel as if you're putting on fresh clothes even if you repeat your jackets and skirts. If you have plans for some evenings out or suspect you will, include at least one dressy blouse or sweater that works with your skirts. It will create a new mood for nighttime and give you a psychological lift.

Unless you are traveling during the summer, you will probably require a coat. Look for one that is lightweight and easy to carry, won't weigh you down when you're wearing it and won't wrinkle easily. A coat that can be worn for rainy days and cool, dry days as well as dressy evenings is ideal, and such coats do exist. For example, choose a rubberized or polyurethane coat that looks great and repels water. Many of these come in dark colors such as black or navy and are elegant enough to wear at night. There are also silk and nylon shells which can be worn on their own or over a cloth or fur coat. If you are traveling in very cold weather, a fur-lined coat is ideal—warm enough to keep you comfortable, dressy without being showy. The key to a good coat is making sure it is long enough to cover your longest skirt or dress.

If there is a possibility that you might have some free time, or if you will be away over a weekend, bring along at least one leisure outfit. This may be a favorite sweater and pants, a pair of jeans or a nifty dress. You'll feel good if you can change from business clothes to something more relaxed when you get in after a hard day. If you bring pants for a day off, consider taking trousers which can also be worn with a dressy top in the evening. Likewise if you are bringing a dress, pack one that can double for dinner too.

One of the benefits of a Travel Capsule is the minimal number of accessories it requires. Instead of endless numbers of shoes and handbags, two pairs of shoes and one or two handbags are all you need. This saves space in your suitcase and keeps it light as well. If you're going to be away for a few days, bring several scarves to enhance your clothes. The addition of a bright-colored bow to a blouse can change the look of an entire outfit. Earrings and necklaces can accomplish a similar effect. If you wear a tailored suit during the day, add earrings and a strand of pearls to it at night to dress it up and make it more feminine.

Three Travel Capsules follow which will keep you well-dressed for at least a week away—one for the Corporate, one for the Communicator and one for the Creative woman. Each one uses black plus another color. You may choose gray or navy instead of the black as any dark color will do.

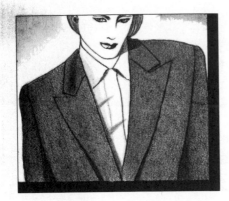

C O R P O R A T E
T R A V E L
C A P S U L E :
B L A C K / B E I G E

As a Corporate woman you may have frequent meetings out of town. You may have to establish rather quickly your power and authority with people you haven't met before. One of the most effective ways to do that, of course, is with your clothes. The twelve pieces in this Capsule include *two jackets, three skirts, one pair of pants, five blouses and one sweater.*

This Travel Capsule is based on *black and beige.* Black is an excellent color for sending a message of authority, and it looks elegant for both day and evening. Beige is used because it is also authoritative, yet lightens the look of some of the outfits. Beige is also sophisticated enough to look smart in the evening. Since in the course of one trip, the Corporate woman may move from city to city and to different climates, this Capsule includes both a light and a dark color.

There are twelve components to pack, and each one yields at least three different looks. The first piece is a black double-breasted jacket. To create a matched suit look include a black straight skirt. The second jacket is a beige and black tweed cardigan style. It too has a matching tweed skirt. The tweed jacket is also worn with the black skirt and the tweed skirt with the black jacket. This gives you four matched or coordinated suit looks. For even more flexibility, include a beige skirt in a silky fabric that can be worn with both jackets.

There are five blouses in this Capsule, all of which are in silky fabrics that look dressy for day and evening. There are two white blouses, each with a convertible collar; a black blouse with a jewel neckline and detachable bow; a shirt style in beige which can be teamed with the beige skirt to make a dress look; and a complementary blouse in an accent color of rust. The rust blouse can relieve the boredom of constantly wearing the same colors and also adds vitality to your appearance. All five of the blouses can be worn with either the black skirt or the tweed skirt and under either of the jackets.

To give another mood to this Capsule, include a pair of black trousers which can be worn for casual occasions such as sightseeing or shopping as well as in the evening. The last piece is a black cardigan sweater which can be worn with the pants, or with either the black skirt or the beige skirt for a different look during the day or at night. The twelve pieces of this Corporate Travel Capsule provide you with looks that range from authoritative to elegantly casual. The pieces include:

- ☐ Black jacket
- ☐ Black and beige tweed jacket
- ☐ Black skirt
- ☐ Black and beige tweed skirt
- ☐ Beige skirt
- ☐ Two white blouses
- ☐ Beige blouse
- ☐ Black blouse
- ☐ Rust blouse
- ☐ Black trousers
- ☐ Black cardigan sweater

Work around the black and beige for your accessories as well. Choose two pairs of shoes in different styles, in black or a black and beige two-tone look. One black leather handbag, preferably an envelope, clutch or neat shoulder bag that can slip inside your attaché, is best. Include a black leather belt, gold and pearl earrings and necklaces, and interesting scarves for your Capsule of accessories.

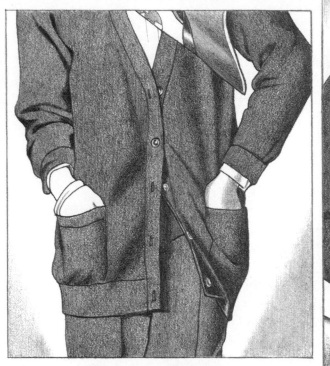
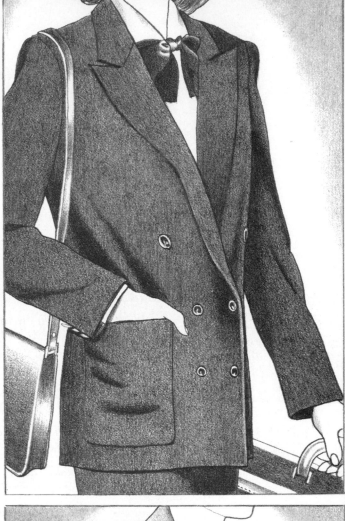
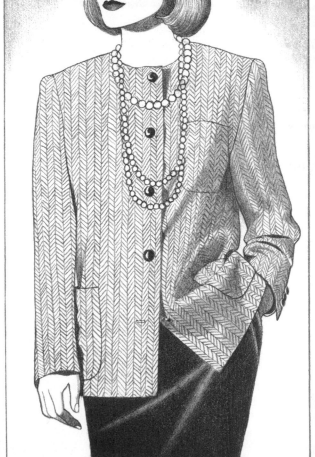
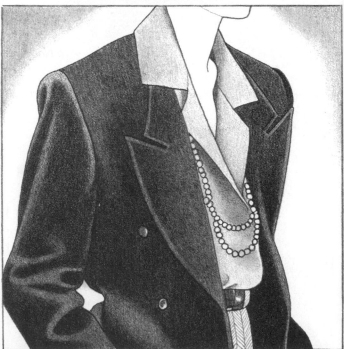

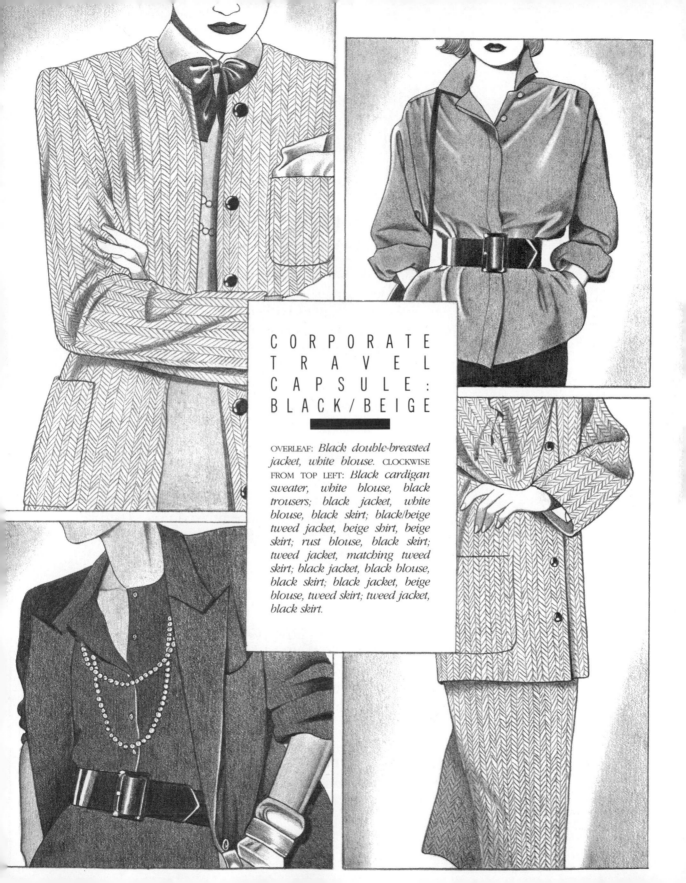

CORPORATE TRAVEL CAPSULE: BLACK/BEIGE

OVERLEAF: *Black double-breasted jacket, white blouse.* CLOCKWISE FROM TOP LEFT: *Black cardigan sweater, white blouse, black trousers; black jacket, white blouse, black skirt; black/beige tweed jacket, beige shirt, beige skirt; rust blouse, black skirt; tweed jacket, matching tweed skirt; black jacket, black blouse, black skirt; black jacket, beige blouse, tweed skirt; tweed jacket, black skirt.*

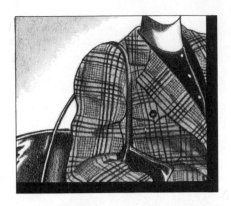

COMMUNICATOR TRAVEL CAPSULE: BLACK/RED

As a Communicator you may attend many different types of events on a ten-day business trip. There may be meetings, speeches, interviews and sales presentations packed into your week away. You may need looks that imply power or suggest affability. It is important to include some clothes that send a message of authority and efficiency as well as other clothes that are softer and more relaxed.

For the Communicator we built a twelve piece Travel Capsule using *black and red* as the base colors. There are *two jackets, two skirts, two dresses, four blouses, one sweater and one pair of pants.* For an authoritative outfit, there is a red jacket piped with black. A black straight skirt is used to tie in with the jacket. This outfit has the power look of a suit with the added energy of the red color.

A second jacket is in a black and red plaid. Again, this has authority but the pattern lends a friendlier, more relaxed note. The plaid jacket works with the black skirt. There is also a soft dirndl skirt in the same plaid that creates a matched suit look.

This Capsule includes two dresses, one in black and the other in red. The black dress is in a long-sleeve shirt style with a detachable white collar and white cuffs. When worn with the collar and cuffs it has a crisp look to it. Worn without the white trim it takes on a completely different look and can be dressed up or down depending upon the occasion. The red dress is in a jumper style; it can be worn for day with a blouse underneath, or dressed up for evening by wearing it without a blouse but with some jewelry or a scarf. Both dresses can be worn alone or with either the red jacket or the plaid jacket.

There are four blouses in this travel group. The first is a white blouse with a detachable bow. It completes the crisp picture of the red jacket and black skirt. It also goes well with the plaid jacket and the black skirt, or can be worn under the red jumper. The second blouse is in a gold tone in a bow neck style. It too works with the red jacket and black skirt, giving it a bolder look. It works as well with the plaid jacket and black skirt and under the red jumper. The third blouse is another white one with a roll collar to create a different effect. The last blouse is in black in a jewel neck style with a detachable scarf. This goes with all of the outfits and can look very dressy in the evening when worn with the black skirt and without a jacket. A similar dressy effect can be created by combining either of the white blouses with the black skirt and using the black scarf or jewelry as accessories.

For times when you go out but are not working, include a bright blue sweater and a pair of black pants. The blue color brings relief from the red and the black, and the sweater adds a casual note. The pants can be worn with the sweater or with any of the blouses. They are great for relaxed times or for dressy occasions in the evening. The twelve pieces in this Communicator Travel Capsule are:

- ☐ Red jacket
- ☐ Black and red plaid jacket
- ☐ Black skirt
- ☐ Black and red plaid skirt
- ☐ Black dress
- ☐ Red dress
- ☐ Two white blouses
- ☐ Black blouse
- ☐ Gold blouse
- ☐ Blue sweater
- ☐ Black pants

The accessories for this Capsule can be kept to a minimum. Two pairs of shoes, preferably both in black, are enough. They go with all of your outfits for day or evening. Choose one low-heeled pump and the other a slightly higher-heeled style. One black handbag is all you need, especially if you use a portfolio, attaché or briefcase and your handbag is small enough to fit inside. This compact purse should be just the right size to use in the evening as well. One black leather belt will go with everything. For jewelry, take along two pairs of earrings— one pearl, the other gold—and the same for necklaces. One or two scarves in red, yellow or bright blue complete the picture.

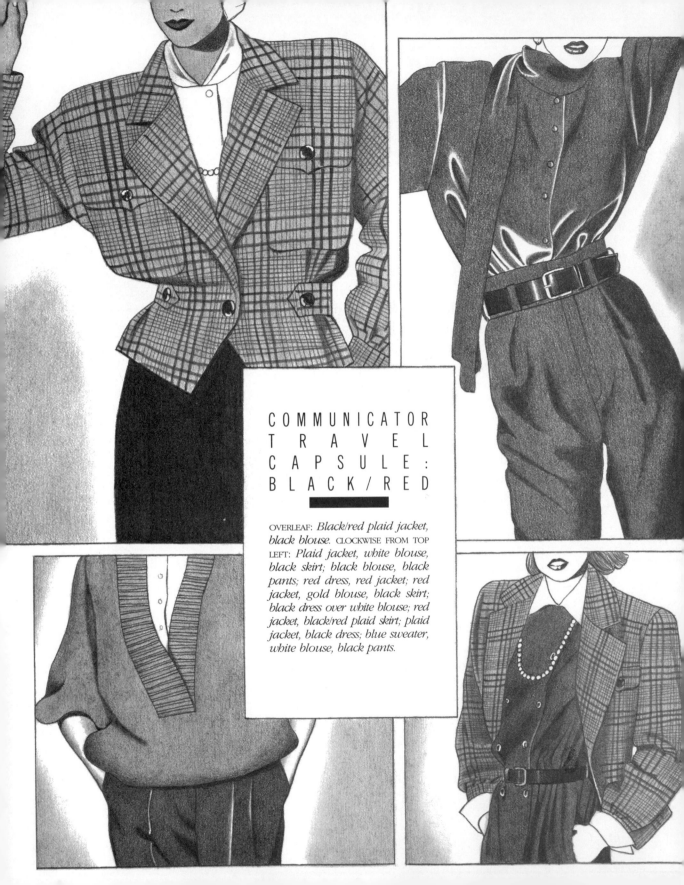

COMMUNICATOR TRAVEL CAPSULE: BLACK/RED

OVERLEAF: *Black/red plaid jacket, black blouse.* CLOCKWISE FROM TOP LEFT: *Plaid jacket, white blouse, black skirt; black blouse, black pants; red dress, red jacket; red jacket, gold blouse, black skirt; black dress over white blouse; red jacket, black/red plaid skirt; plaid jacket, black dress; blue sweater, white blouse, black pants.*

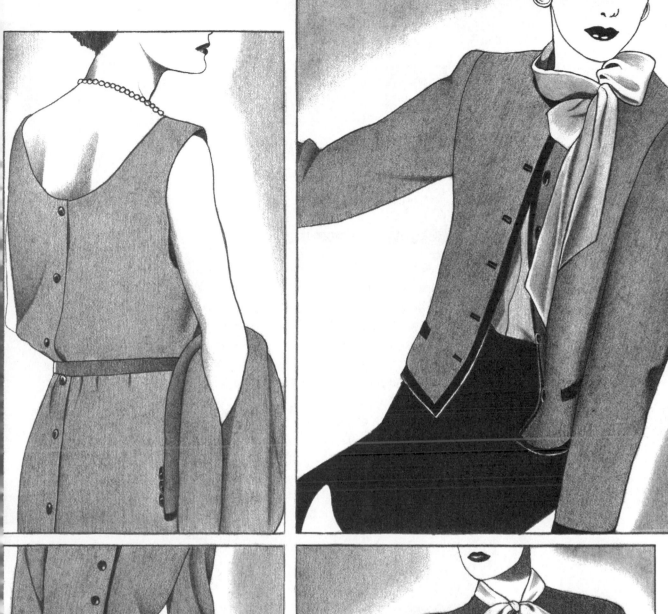
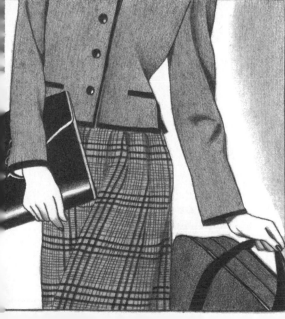
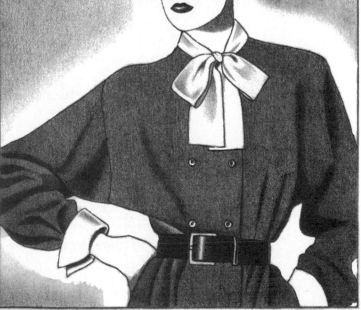

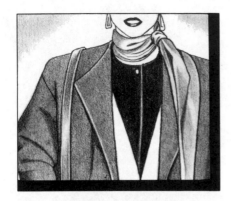

The third Travel Capsule is for the Creative woman. You may take a five day trip with just seven items. Like your Corporate and Communicator colleagues, use black as one of the base colors but combine it with white for a striking effect. There is *one skirt, one pair of pants, three blouses, one sweater and one jacket.*

In this group, we have one black skirt and one pair of black pants. With them pack a long-sleeve white blouse in a convertible collar shirt style which can be worn open or closed; a second blouse in black in a long-sleeve, jewel neck, button-front style which can be worn as a blouse or over the white shirt as a jacket; a white tunic which can be worn over both the skirt and the pants; and a black turtleneck sweater which can be worn alone or under the white blouse, the black blouse, or the white tunic. The last component in this group is a jacket in brilliant purple to go with everything. This multi-mood Capsule includes:

- ☐ Black skirt
- ☐ Black pants
- ☐ White blouse
- ☐ Black jewel neck blouse
- ☐ White tunic
- ☐ Black turtleneck sweater
- ☐ Purple jacket

As a Creative woman choose a few unusual accessories to complement your Travel Capsule. You too can manage with just two pairs of black shoes, but the styles can be more high-fashion than your colleagues may select. One black handbag, a small purse and a large tote or portfolio for papers are adequate. For belts, take a bright red leather one, or a black leather belt with a handtooled buckle. Jewelry might include a few bold pieces in earrings, and a necklace. One or two scarves, in red, purple, black or a vibrant print, will suffice.

Any of these three Travel Capsules fits easily into either a hanging garment bag or a suitcase. Since luggage is often misplaced or delayed by airlines, many people are finding it easier to travel with carry-on luggage only, preferably a hanging bag. If you don't have one already, look for a hanging bag that has roomy pockets on the back and is long enough to hold your skirts and dresses. Fortunately, hanging bags are now being made for women. These are longer than the men's styles and will keep your clothes from getting creased. The back pockets are handy for storing blouses, accessories, intimate apparel, a hand steamer, electric rollers, and your cosmetics kit. Shoes can be put in the front and will fall to the bottom, out of the way of your clothes.

If you prefer a suitcase, those made of a lightweight material, such as canvas, are a good idea for the times you have to carry it yourself. Although some women are using carrying wheels, these can give you a false sense of security. They have been known to fall off midway to the airline terminal leaving their owners with suitcases that are too heavy or too clumsy to carry. They are also cumbersome and can cause ill will among fellow passengers when you are getting on and off the airplane. For a short trip consider using a suitcase that fits under your airplane seat. These bags are large enough to hold a change of clothes, cosmetics and sleepwear yet small enough for you to carry on board.

When packing a suitcase, use your shoes, jewelry roll, electric curlers, hand steamer and other solid items to line the sides and keep your clothes from sliding around inside. Use tissue paper to stuff sleeves and as a layer between clothes to keep them from wrinkling. The clear plastic bags used by dry cleaners also prevent wrinkles if you use them between each layer of clothing; they can also serve to separate your laundry on the trip home.

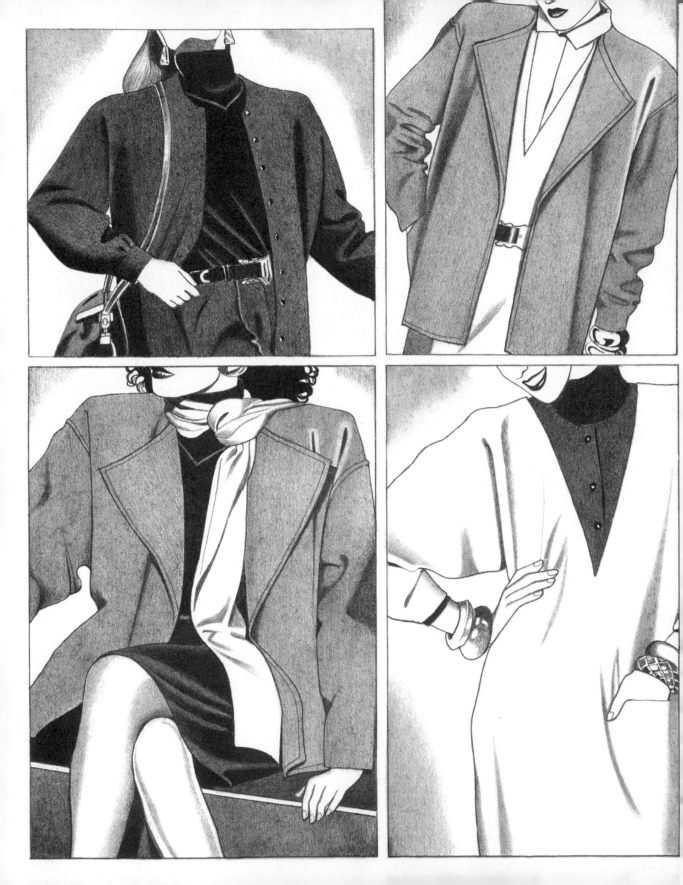

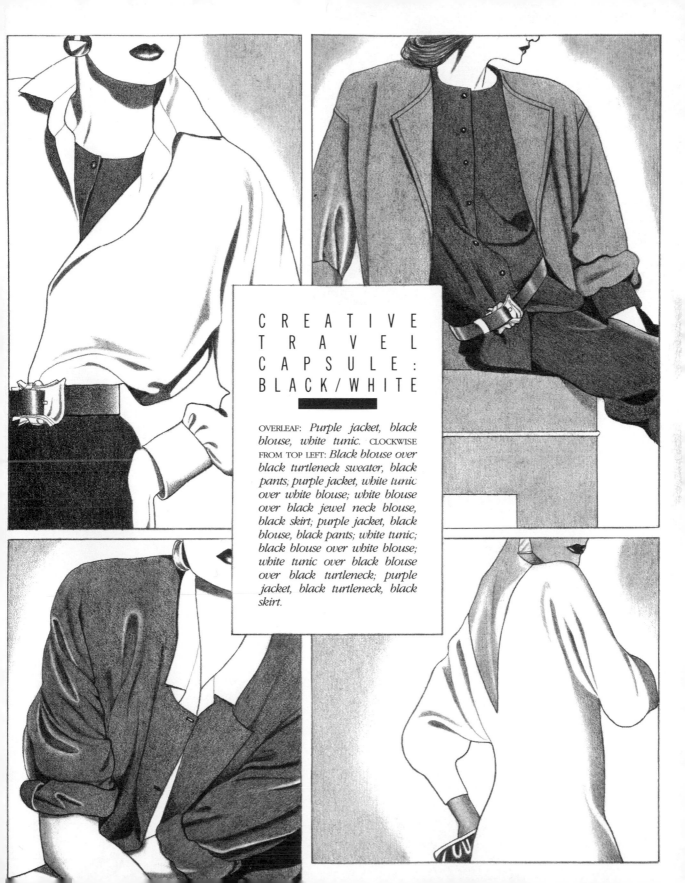

CREATIVE TRAVEL CAPSULE: BLACK/WHITE

OVERLEAF: *Purple jacket, black blouse, white tunic.* CLOCKWISE FROM TOP LEFT: *Black blouse over black turtleneck sweater, black pants; purple jacket, white tunic over white blouse; white blouse over black jewel neck blouse, black skirt; purple jacket, black blouse, black pants; white tunic; black blouse over white blouse; white tunic over black blouse over black turtleneck; purple jacket, black turtleneck, black skirt.*

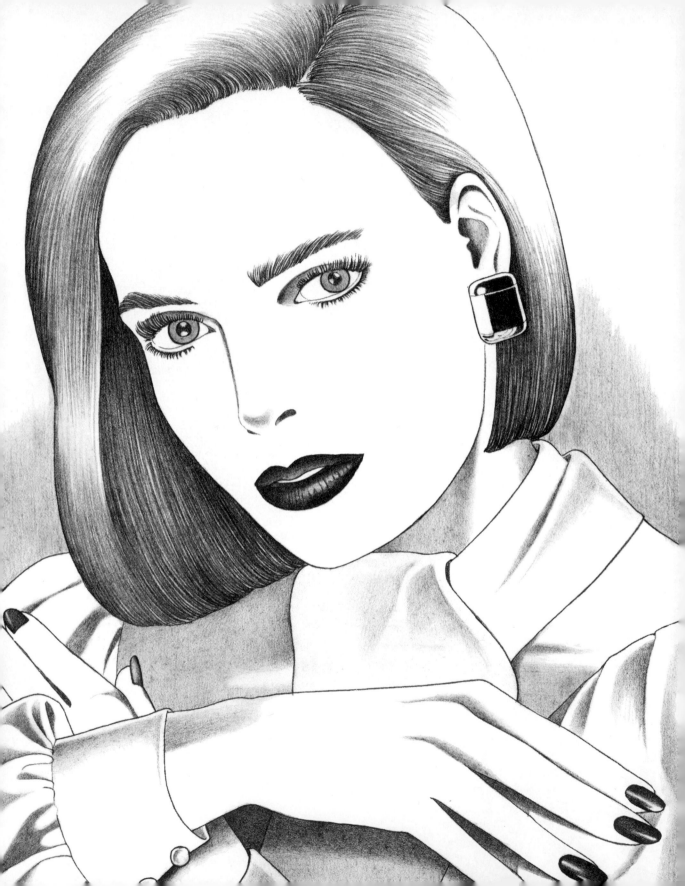

CHAPTER XIII

Good Grooming: A Guide to Skin and Hair Care

One of the most striking features of many successful women is their impeccable grooming: not just clothes, but hair, makeup, and hands are all in perfect order. Whether or not they have natural good looks or great figures, their spruced-up appearance helps them stand apart and gives them an air of self-assurance that overcomes any weak features or figure faults.

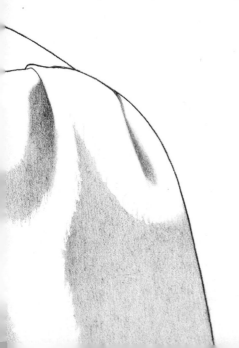

Think of some women who stand out in their fields: Dianne Feinstein and Elizabeth Dole in politics; Helen Gurley Brown in publishing; Geraldine Stutz in retailing; Mary Wells Lawrence in advertising; Diane Sawyer in television. Despite overloaded schedules, each of them manages to include a beauty routine that keeps them looking polished. Their hair is always in place, their makeup always in order, their nails manicured, and their clothes clean and pressed. They look self-confident and self-possessed.

Francesco Scavullo has photographed the beautiful and famous from Racquel Welch to Diana Ross to Nancy Reagan. When he talks about attractive women, he refers to their good grooming rather than their great looks. "I love a woman that's neat and looks very clean," he says. Scavullo describes Nancy Reagan this way: "She has clean, beautifully-cut hair. Her skin looks beautiful."

That old adage "neatness counts" matters more than you may think. An impeccable appearance says that your work habits are also impeccable. It is an indication of your organizational strengths (you must be well-organized if you both manage a career and keep yourself well-groomed); your self-discipline; and your attention to details. An appearance that is neat and precise is a strong indication that you don't slide over things and are attentive to specifics. Good grooming is to your appearance what good diction is to public speaking: If you dress and look precise, you send a message that you are precise, you are efficient, and that you think before you act.

This is not to suggest that you ought to be obsessed with taking care of yourself. Doing your nails at your desk or repairing your makeup during a meeting is not only inappropriate, it's bad manners. No one wants to watch you grooming yourself. These personal details should be attended to far away from the office. It is also not a subject to be discussed on business time. Talking about hair, makeup, nails or clothing in the workplace detracts from the perception of you as a professional woman. At the same time, looking attractive will help you vis-à-vis your audience.

Mary Wells Lawrence said at the *Vogue* symposium, "People like women to look as though they can afford to dress nicely, that they take good care of themselves, that they are very clean, that they take time to get their hair done regularly, that they do makeup fairly well, that they know what's going on in the fashion world. That they're not boring."

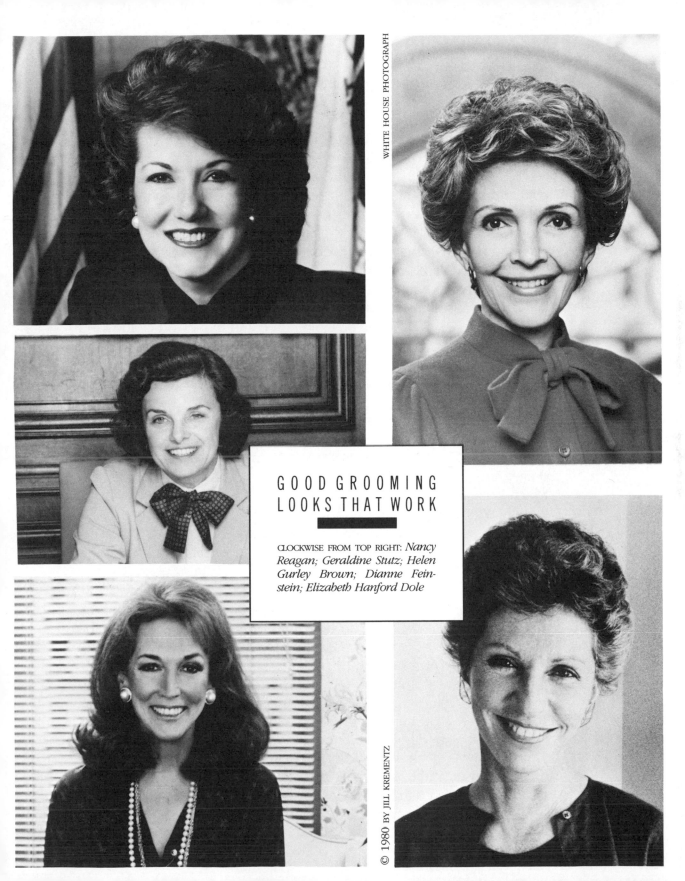

GOOD GROOMING LOOKS THAT WORK

CLOCKWISE FROM TOP RIGHT: *Nancy Reagan; Geraldine Stutz; Helen Gurley Brown; Dianne Feinstein; Elizabeth Hanford Dole*

It does take some planning to be well-groomed, but it is well worth the extra effort. For some women, a beauty regimen early in the morning is ideal; for others late nights or weekends are the best times. When I worked as fashion director for Garfinckel's, I often traveled with another woman whose body clock was the opposite of mine. She would get up at six in the morning to wash her hair, set it, give herself a manicure and so on. I admired her ability to rise so early but I needed my morning sleep too much to do the same. Instead, I was willing to spend a few hours late at night taking care of my needs. As you set a routine for yourself, be realistic. The best regime will only work if you set up a schedule based on your body clock.

No matter how much time you devote to your clothes, you won't be properly dressed unless your makeup and hairstyle are done with care too. There's no point in spending time and money on clothes and then leaving your face and hair to chance. No fashion designer would have mannequins wear his clothes without their makeup and hairstyle as finished as the outfits. It's all part of the total package. It would be wonderful if women could get by without makeup, but for most of us, the reality is that we look more attractive when we use skin treatments and cosmetics.

In the business and professional world, war paint is inappropriate, nor does a bare face work either. The most winning look is one which is clean, fresh and natural. But it takes more than nature to make it happen.

SKIN CARE

QUICK CLEANSING ROUTINE. Before you think about makeup, consider the kind of skin you have and the best way to clean it. Makeup must be applied to clean skin. Otherwise, you are only covering the dirt and intensifying any problems you may have. Says Marianne Dorio of Prescriptives, "The first thing to look at is your skin condition. Covering up and altering features is not the contemporary way to do things. Ask yourself: How can I improve my skin so my makeup will make me look my best self—not different than I really am."

Whether their skin is dry or oily, most women use soap and water cleanser. Although this feels cleaner, it may dry out your skin, making it feel taut and look flaky.

If you have dry skin, use soap or a cleansing lather that has an emollient to protect your skin from losing its natural oils. One treatment that helps keep dry skin looking smooth is exfoliation. This sounds drastic but it is simply an easy way to slough off dead skin. Many skin treatment lines include exfoliants. There are also special cotton washcloths made with a slightly rough surface that acts to scrub off dead skin cells. Using an exfoliant while you are taking your shower in the morning is an effective way to open the pores and clean away the dead cells. Prescriptives has an exfoliator with a mild clay base that contains granules of mineral oil. Always follow up the cleansing with a moisturizer to replenish your skin with oils and minerals. One New York socialite who has an exquisite complexion (and who can afford the most expensive cosmetics) uses Crisco to moisturize her skin.

If you have oily skin, use a soap and water cleansing routine twice a day. Apply an astringent after cleansing to remove excess oil. If your face is very oily, you may find it helpful to apply astringent during the day to soak up the oils. A facial mask for oily skin will act as a mild exfoliant while tightening the pores. Since you want to keep your pores from enlarging, use a facial mask while you are in the shower; it will clean away dead skin cells while tightening your pores. Orlane has a mild facial mask that can be used every day. Adrienne Arpel makes a sea mud pack that is stronger and very effective. Even if you have oily skin, you may need to follow up with a light moisturizer, particularly in sensitive areas such as under the eyes.

Several cosmetics firms have skin treatment regimens for various skin conditions. Erno Laszlo, Clinique, and Janet Sartin have soap and water regimens based on skin types from very dry to very oily. Laszlo's soap for oily skin contains sea mud minerals, while his routine for dry skin includes a pre-treatment oil. Laszlo also has conditioning preparations such as a controlling lotion for oily skin, a moisture retention lotion for dry skin, and a light moisturizer for people with combination skin. One way to find out more about skin products is to talk to the consultants behind the counter. Even better, ask friends or acquaintances. I learned about Laszlo by asking a colleague how her skin condition had improved so dramatically. She was delighted to tell me about her new routine. Most people are pleased to share their information with you.

A good cleansing shouldn't take more than a few minutes. Like any routine, once you are used to the steps, it is quick and efficient.

MAKEUP

FOUNDATION. Now you can begin thinking about cosmetics. The first step is your foundation, which should be linked to your cleansing treatment. If your skin is dry, use a foundation which contains an oil base. This acts as a moisturizer as well as protection for your skin. If you have oily skin, use a foundation that has a water base; an emollient may just aggravate the condition.

A foundation gives you a smooth finish. It is the best base for applying color to cheeks, eyes and lips and helps colors stay on longer. It also acts as an outer layer and protects your bare skin from the elements: cold, dry, wind, soot and pollution.

If the foundation you have been using feels heavy, it may be too rich for your skin. Look for one that is lighter, perhaps with less oil. If the color is wrong, you can really look as if you are wearing a mask. It is best to have a foundation that matches your skin tone rather than one that contrasts. You don't want to be in a meeting or making a presentation, and find that everyone is staring at the orange line at your jaw.

The best way to discover the correct color for your face is to try a stroke of foundation on the bare skin at your jaw line. This is the true color of your skin. (Very often at cosmetic counters salespeople will test foundation on your hand, but this skin is rarely the same color as your face.) Skin colors tend to either a red, yellow, or blue undertone. As you apply different foundation shades, you'll see which one blends in best with your own skin tones.

FIVE MINUTE MAKEUP. Your everyday makeup routine can be quick and easy. Experiment with new colors, new looks in your spare time. Use the following checklist for daily application.

- Before applying any color to your face, use a translucent powder over your foundation. This sets the base and helps it last longer.
- Put on cheek color—just enough to look natural—and powder the cheek to help the color stay.

- Next, do your eyes the same way: first with foundation, then translucent powder, then eye shadow, and powder. Use subtle rather than bright colors to enhance your eyes. (White rimmed, owlish eyes can be very disconcerting. If you use a concealer under your eyes, be sure to blend it very well with your foundation.)
- Liner, above and below the eyes, can help accentuate them. Follow with a coating of mascara in brown or black, first on the top, then underneath the lashes. Don't forget the lashes closer to the inside of your eye as well as the lower lashes.
- The last step is color on your lips. A lip pencil is effective for setting a clean line. To keep the outline from looking harsh, use a pencil in the same color as your lipstick. If you fill in your lips with the pencil, you'll have a base of color that stays on most of the day. Then cover with lipstick for a rich coating. To achieve a moist look, add lip gloss over your lipstick. This whole routine should not take more than five minutes.

COSMETICS BASICS

Just as you have a Capsule of clothes, you should have a Capsule of cosmetics. Besides your one foundation, include two blushers, one in the red or orange family and one in the pink family; two lipsticks, one to go with reds or oranges, the other to go with pinks; and at least one eye shadow.

Sometimes women seem to disintegrate during the day. They start out in the morning looking great, then lose their makeup as the day wears on. Keep translucent powder in your desk or purse. Apply it during the day to keep your makeup looking fresh.

There are also special tools that are efficient time savers. Cosmetics brushes can be a big help in applying makeup. They are often sold in sets that include a large brush for loose powder, a smaller brush for blending eye shadows, an eyebrow brush, a mascara comb, and a lip brush. A makeup sponge can also be effective for blending your foundation.

For touch-ups in public, make sure you use an attractive compact and lipstick.

If you use nail color, keep a supply in your desk. You may need to repair your nails if the color chips.

HAND CARE

Shaking hands is an integral and important part of meeting people. In addition, you use your hands when you speak or make a presentation. If you are involved in selling a product, imagine how much better it displays if you show it with attractive hands. Your hands represent an important part of your appearance, not just to see but to touch as well.

Hands that are cared for reflect well on their owner. This means not just filing your nails and applying polish, but a regimen of hand care. To start, protect your hands by using a hand cream. This also makes your hands pleasant to touch when you shake hands with someone. If you spend a fair amount of time outdoors in the hot sun and are susceptible to sunspots, use a sunscreen or a hand cream that contains a sunscreen in order to keep your hands from looking prematurely aged. Massage your hands with cream in the morning and at night. Keep some hand cream in your desk and if your hands feel dry or chafed, apply the cream to the back and gently rub your hands back to back.

FIFTEEN-MINUTE MANICURE. As part of your grooming regimen, give yourself a complete manicure once a week. If you wear nail polish, remove it gently with nail polish remover. Polish remover is strong stuff and can harm the surface of your nails, so don't overdo it.

Shape your nails with a fine emery board using the smooth side. File them towards the center. If you file them back and forth you'll cause them to break. Long, pointy nails are inappropriate for work, particularly if you are a Corporate woman. Keep them short and nicely rounded. Then buff the surface of your nails with a buffer. This will smooth them out if you have any splits or cracks.

Next, soak your fingers in warm, soapy water to soften the cuticles. Then apply cuticle oil or cream and gently push back the cuticles with a special cuticle stick. Don't cut your cuticles with a scissors as this can cause an infection; use a cuticle scissors to carefully cut away hangnails.

Now massage in hand cream. The massage will soften your hands after being in the water and also help the circulation in your hands and nails. Dry off any excess cream.

Applying polish is the trickiest part. First, use a clear base. This acts like a foundation to protect the nails and hold the polish better. For a long-lasting manicure, use two coats of base. Always make sure the first coat is dry before applying the second coat, otherwise the polish will not dry properly and will be more likely to peel.

After the base coats, apply a color. Because strong colors can be distracting and difficult to maintain, consider a soft color or even clear polish. These will not require the touch-ups that bright color does. Save strong reds for the evening. If you have short nails, bright color will just make your hands look stubby, while lighter shades will make your hands look longer. Apply two coats of polish. This will last longer and even strengthen your nails. When the polish dries, apply a clear top coat to seal the color and give your nails a finished look. If the polish chips and you have to reapply color during the week, first apply base to the tips, then add a coat of color and a coat of sealer.

HAIR CARE

"If there is one specific thing that comes across, it's being well-groomed and having clean, fresh hair," says New York hairstylist Leslie Blanchard. "That shows a person cares about themselves. If they take an interest in themselves, then everyone they're working with knows they take more of an interest in what they're doing." With clients like Barbara Walters, Meryl Streep and Mary Tyler Moore, and with his own frequent television appearances around the country, Blanchard is tuned in to the needs of working women. Above everything, he emphasizes clean, bouncy hair. Here are some of his recommendations for hair treatment, cut and style.

Stress, activity and pollution can play havoc. You may need to wash your hair as often as every day. Tension cuts off circulation, and washing your hair is good stimulation for the scalp. If you are very active, involved in exercise programs or athletics, there is a perspiration buildup that requires frequent shampooing.

Although many women are concerned that shampooing may harm their hair, it won't if followed with a conditioner, even one that is rinsed out. If your hair has been chemically treated or if you use hot rollers or a blow dryer, however, use a conditioner that stays in the hair. This will give it a better sheen.

CUT AND SHAPE. Foremost, get a good haircut. A good cut should hold a set, keep its shape, and give you at least two different ways to wear your hair. Very fashionable hairstyles may look great in the evening but are inappropriate for day. A good cut allows you to style your hair both for work and nighttime.

Although there is a wide range of women's hairstyles, there are preferred looks for each profile. The Corporate woman should keep her hair to a moderate length, preferably not below the chin. Wear your hair away from your face to keep it from being distracting. If your hair is long, pull it back during the daytime into a neat knot. The Communicator should also keep her hairstyle simple and no longer than shoulder length. Although it doesn't have to be quite as efficient looking, it should always be neat. Too many curls or too much frizz takes away from a well-groomed look, but avoid anything too stiff as this may suggest a rigid personality.

Proportion is very important. Take a look at your whole self in a full-length mirror: If you are small, a lot of hair will seem overwhelming; if you are tall, very short hair can look ridiculous. There should be a balance between the length of your hair and your overall height and size. A cropped cut tends to make a woman look masculine. Very long hair, on the other hand, takes away from a business or professional attitude. Your hairstyle should also be appropriate to your age. Hair that hangs below the shoulder generally looks inappropriate on older women. Younger women should be careful not to choose anything too severe.

One way to change your look is with gels and mousses. Gels give your hair a wet, glossy look, more useful for the Creative woman than the Corporate or Communicator types. Mousses make the hair easier to mold, and can be helpful for shaping your hair into style. Think of mousse as a light setting lotion.

Even the best hairstyle usually needs a light hairspray to keep it in place. One of the favorites of many models is Final Net's extra-hold version.

COLOR. In a survey among executives, conducted for Blanchard, it was found that most people perceive blondes and brunettes to be equally capable. But dark-haired women were considered to be more authoritative, more aggressive, and more decisive than blondes. For the Corporate woman, dark hair is definitely an asset. Blondes, however, were perceived as being friendlier and more popular, excellent attributes for the Communicator. If you are changing fields, bear in mind that your hair color does affect other people's perception of you. It can also have an impact on the way you feel about yourself. If you are making a career change, you may want to change your hair color and your hairstyle at the same time. But if you decide to change your hair color while in the same job, do it slowly, in stages; both you and your colleagues will find it easier to adjust.

Always take your natural color into consideration. Your hair tone should always blend with your skin tone: If you have reddish undertones in your face, choose a hair color that has the same cast; if your skin is yellowish, your hair color should have a similar undertone. Hair coloring is not damaging to the hair. It makes it more manageable, gives it more body.

There are three different methods you can use to color your hair. The first is a semi-permanent color that gradually shampoos away. It is a good color enhancer which gives a gloss to your hair. This rinse is an easy method to cover gray until your hair is at least 10 percent gray, when you might consider a longer lasting technique.

The second process is highlighting. This is excellent for enhancing your natural color. As your own hair color changes, keep the highlighting colors relating harmoniously.

The third method is permanent hair coloring. If you have a good deal of gray hair and want to color it, this is the best technique. It is precise and you can achieve the exact color you want. But this method requires constant follow-up and should be done on a regular basis every four or five weeks.

There are many women who look extremely attractive with naturally gray hair. As your hair becomes more gray, you may have to adjust your makeup. You'll find that colors—both makeup and clothing—look different on you; some of the shades you never wore before may now look terrific.

TIPS. Here are twelve quick tips for your hair from Blanchard:

1. Always shampoo your hair in the morning to give it the most shine and bounce during the day.
2. Never go to bed with wet hair. If you sleep on your hair before it is totally dry, it will be bent out of shape in the morning.
3. Do not sleep on curlers or rollers. They can cause permanent damage to the hair and scalp, weaken the hair's roots and embed a pattern in your hair.
4. Never get a haircut from a hairdresser the first time you go to the salon. First talk to the stylist and see what he or she suggests. Make sure you're on the same wavelength before you let them take up the scissors. Look around at the other customers. If you wear your hair long, and all the other clients have short hair, this may not be the salon for you.
5. When you have your hair cut, make sure you can have at least two or three different looks with it.
6. If you use electric curlers or blow dryers constantly, then shampoo and condition every day as protective measures.
7. Brushing your hair 100 times a day is not a good idea; it can make your hair oily.
8. Washing your hair does not dry it out. If your hair tends to be dry or oily, is color treated, or fragile, look for appropriate products to correct these conditions.
9. If you have flyaway hair, put some kind of cream over it for extra control.

10. Always read labels. If there is oil in a product, it will attract soil and dirt.
11. Hairsprays should give you control, not stiffness. Your hair should not look as if it will break with a chisel and hammer.
12. Don't be intimidated by a hairdresser. If you are, move on fast to somebody else.

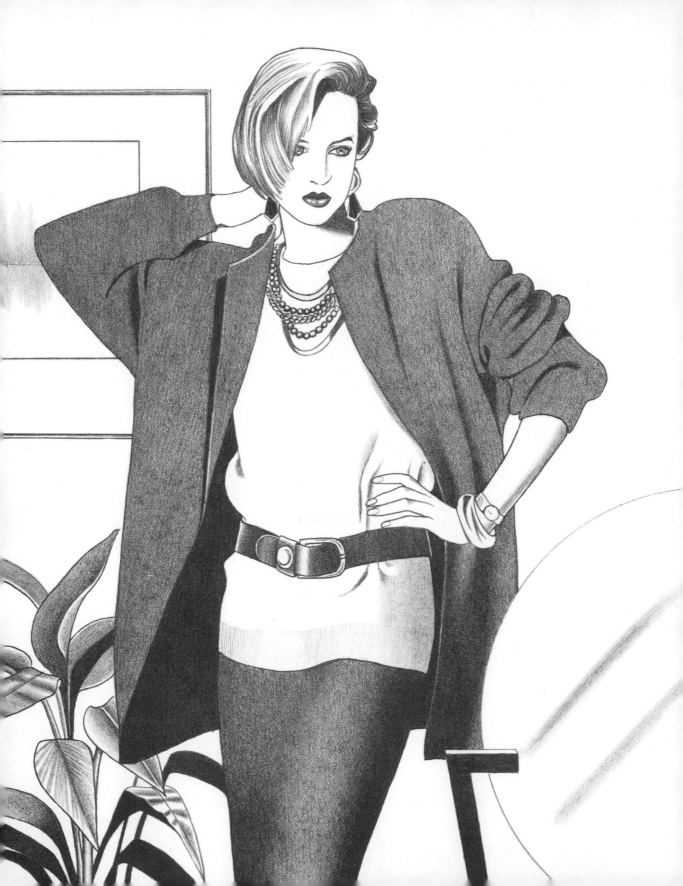

CHAPTER XIV

The Elements of Style

Whatever your career profile, let your personal style shine through. The stronger your stamp the greater your visibility, and the easier your identification within your organization. You can stay within the framework of your profile—whether Corporate, Communicator, or Creative—play by the rules, and still cultivate your own style. A strong sense of personal style emphasizes that you have confidence in yourself; it indicates that you have strong career potential, that you are a leader, not a follower.

Jean Sisco is an influential business consultant who sees dressing as a tool in career strategy. She is an articulate woman who communicates accomplishment in her speech, her body language and her appearance. She is concerned about women who melt into the background.

She says, "I think part of this goes with the training of a woman . . . you don't make yourself stand out, you don't laugh too loudly, you blend; you become a more passive person. I think women try to select their dress to conform to this passivity. *They make themselves bland by attempting to blend.* Consequently, it totally detracts from any feeling of authority, from a successful projection of image, from really being able to take a lead."

On a more positive note, Sisco says she does see more and more women paying attention to their appearance. "I am so delighted when I go into a corporation, either as a consultant or a director, and I see the women adding a little color and vitality and spark. You can be very businesslike and yet you can introduce color and style notes and good line and design that do not distract."

Sisco believes that visibility is becoming more and more of a factor in the daily agenda of working women; and the bottom line is that the way women appear on the various and diverse occasions during a business week makes a difference. Says Sisco, "No business comes easy anymore. The first thing that comes across is how you appear. Frankly, a woman's appearance is far more important than a man's. Not fair, but absolutely important. It doesn't have to be anything too strident. Too blatant, too overdone is wrong. But you definitely should not be a non-entity."

Adrienne Feldman is an effective, attractive attorney who made this observation about a woman lawyer she met: "Her whole self was without crispness. Her hair just hung there. It was as if there was a woman underneath who would love to wear a hat and look stylish but somewhere along the line wasn't willing to commit herself. If you make a statement with your clothes that you are stylish, you hold yourself up for expectation, if not comment. You are more noticed and have to take more responsibility than if you are without style and hang back."

Your own style may evolve over a period of time. Almost all of us have gone through various fashion stages, from following teen-age fads to testing high-fashion looks. A great deal of striking out on our own clothes-wise has to do with searching for our own identities, and finding ourselves as individuals. The confusion about what we wear is sometimes muddled with our confusion about ourselves or our careers. For some people, it may be easier to choose a role which comes with its own costume. That sets the boundaries and limits the possibilities for mistakes. If you work for an airline or are in the medical profession, the prescribed uniforms make your clothing choices fairly easy. But many women reject the narrow definitions of a uniform. Indeed, for some women, the solutions, at least temporarily, may come in the form of off-beat or even bizarre-looking clothes.

Harriet Hentges worked at the White House under President Jimmy Carter and later for Sears International, a world-wide trading division of Sears Roebuck. But before she embarked on this career path, Harriet was a nun. When she entered the convent at the age of eighteen, the style of dress was still the traditional nun's habit. Although at first it was difficult for her to learn to manage the many layers and yards of material, it didn't take long before she enjoyed the ritual of dressing and the respect her clothing drew. She even rejected the idea of wearing more secular type clothing when the Church moved in that direction. Her identity was wrapped up in her habit.

At about the same time, Dena Sollins was starting her career as a commentator for the Canadian Broadcasting Company. Although her perspective may have been quite different, she too was questioning her own identity and exploring her personality through her style of dressing. She says, "I think that like so many women my age . . . we were reared to be an ornament, in my case, a cultured ornament to a man. And so when I was in my early twenties—that was the time when the women's movement really was at its peak—I knew that a lot of my power was in my looks. I didn't have as much confidence as to what was in my head or in my soul. So I dressed to attract attention, and often that was provocatively, or very bohemian, or in bright colors, or *different*. All that I knew was that I wanted to stand out in a crowd. So that was the way I dressed.

"Then, friends, peers, colleagues were very much involved in the women's movement and I also started to question my values, my body, my appearance—really my identity. What I think happened was, as I got older, I became more comfortable with the person that I was. I became more confident as my career developed, became more confident in my abilities. And I did not feel the need to stand out in the crowd. There was certain joy in the subtlety. I think it was very much a change in my identity."

Although she moved away from the outrageous, she says, "I was still very interested in fashion and style. I was developing, I hope, more style in my character and I think it was reflected in the way that I dressed."

Sollins didn't change overnight. Nor did she then adopt the style of dressing that she has now. "I like elegance, and I'm still very interested in colors and textures. When you work in the arts elegance is all around you, so those tastes were developing at the same time. Now I dress much more classically. I think I've gone through several changes. I think clothes are costumes, and it's so marvelous. Women are lucky."

THREE IMPORTANT POINTS

Whether your career calls for a kind of uniform or more creative clothing, there are several factors to keep in mind when you are dressing.

Since your appearance is a way of sending a message, you might compare it to the way you would write a business letter. Catalyst lists the three most important points of letter writing: "Always speak (or write) in the receiver's language; always be precise when expressing yourself; let your personality come through in your letters." Those same guidelines may be used in dressing.

First, *dress in a way that your audience understands.* For example, if you are an executive addressing a group of financial analysts and you appear before them in avant-garde clothes, or frou-frou or ruffly looks, you'll have to work harder to gain their acceptance. Even if you are a fashion designer or are in some other creative field, you'll be at odds with the financial analysts' usual way of dress. It will take them longer to accept you on their terms than if you dressed in something with which they can identify. For example, if you were to appear before them in a simple dress or elegant suit with an interesting accessory (like a handtooled belt or hand-painted scarf), you would be recognizable. You would be dressing in their language but using your own accent. But if you were to appear in purple suede pants and a red leather jacket, your credibility as someone who understands their concerns would be in doubt. This doesn't mean that you have to dress in a gray flannel suit with a bow at your neck. By all means you have a right, even an obligation as a speaker, to stand out from the crowd. But stand out in a way that says you are like them, but uniquely you, and you'll capture your crowd that much faster. You'll be speaking their language, perhaps a bit more eloquently.

Second, *dress and look precise.* Precision in dressing translates into good grooming. One of the features that stands out among almost all successful women is their emphasis on neatness. Although their clothing may be different and their personal styles may vary, they are well-groomed, look precise. Their hair is cut well and neatly combed, their nails are manicured, their makeup is carefully applied, and, of course, their clothing is clean and well-pressed. This good grooming goes along with an attention to detail that distinguishes the professional from the amateur. Another aspect of dressing and looking precise is to have a look that is pulled together and well-coordinated. If you enjoy wearing accessories, for example, don't overload them. If you like bright colors, choose one to highlight your outfit. Remember that if your audience's eye is pulled from your ears to your neck to your lapel to your waist, you are distracting them from hearing your message.

Third, *let your personality show through in the way you dress.* You may dress in the most conservative kinds of clothes but there is still room for some individuality. For example, you may wear something as basic as a gray flannel suit, but the quality of the cut and the fabric will indicate that you are a person who appreciates good things. You can let your personality show through by the blouse and the accessories that you choose to wear with that suit. The colors, the shapes and the materials all say something about you. Make sure, however, that your message is unified. Too many extras take away from the clarity of your message.

The language you speak may have to be altered slightly from audience to audience. Even the meanings of the words may change. What spells success in one community may spell disaster in another. That is why being aware of your audience's language is so important. One woman who understands this is Communicator Nancy Reynolds. A close friend of President and Mrs. Reagan, Reynolds was in charge of the Washington office of the Bendix Corporation. Now, as a lobbyist for the motion picture industry, she is sharply aware of the symbolism of clothing both in Hollywood and on the east coast. She says that when she invites her film industry clients to testify, "My first admonition is, 'Please don't wear what I saw you in the last time I was out in California.' Flashy kinds of clothes which look fine there are absolutely viewed with suspicion in Washington."

She adds that her clients are not always aware of the language differences. "They always say, 'Why aren't we looked upon with more respect in Washington?' And I answer, 'Because in their eyes you are from LaLa Land. When you come back and don't dress as the natives do, and speak as the natives do, it confirms all their suspicions of, Ah ha, I told you so. Those are rocky people out there'."

The message is clear to Reynolds that success is communicated through the language of the locals. Leather pants and a hand-painted blouse might translate into creativity in Hollywood, but in the nation's capital it means something flaky. And while on Capitol Hill conservative clothing means sincerity, out in Hollywood it is downright dull. So be aware of which language your audience speaks before you address it; at the same time, bear in mind that people admire individuality and flair.

EXPERIMENT WITH DIFFERENT LOOKS

It takes a certain amount of self-confidence to have a personal style, and you can gain that self-confidence by experimenting at home with different looks. You may not feel sure of what is right, or what looks good on you. You may not want to invest a great deal of money in clothes that you are not sure of—nor should you. The wisest way to go about this is to begin with classic clothes, clothes that you know will work for you and will last a long time. From there, you can try out new looks, either in the dressing room of a store or in the privacy of your home. You may test out new colors and fabrics, new accessories, and new shapes.

A small change can have a big effect on your appearance. You'll see that by switching the color of a blouse or the way you wear the collar, you'll change the look of your whole outfit. For example, if you're wearing a suit, try it first with a white cotton blouse, then with a white silk blouse. Then try a blouse in a strong color such as red or blue, and finally try a print blouse with it. Even wearing a collar open or closed, inside your jacket or over your lapels, can make a big difference. Each time you change your blouse, you change the attitude of the outfit.

Try the same thing with accessories. Shoes, for example, can make an enormous difference. Put on a pair of pumps with your suit and then switch to sandals. Change the shoe colors and see how that affects the outfit. Do the same with jewelry. Try a pair of simple pearl or gold earrings. Then try on bright-colored earrings or ones that dangle. As you experiment with these different looks, you'll begin to see what looks best on you and how you would like to look. But keep in mind the parameters of your career profile.

Subtle touches may make the difference. The quality of cut, fit and fabric in higher-priced clothing is usually well worth the extra money. You may never know how wonderful a well-made suit can look until you see it on. Allow yourself the luxury of trying one on. Until you see how a well-cut garment fits you, how it looks, and how it feels, you may not understand the difference it makes. Even though you may not be able to afford it right now, you owe yourself the education of seeing what makes it worth its price tag. (And, at a later date, you may find that same suit or a similar one on sale or at a discount store.) Look at the way it fits your body. Clothes that are made for the mass market must fit tens of thousands of women; the patterns leave enough room for everybody's figure problems. But more expensive clothing is cut for an exclusive few. There is more attention that goes into the pattern-making. Feel the fabric. If it feels soft and light, it has what the professionals call "a good hand." Look at the details: the buttons, the pockets, the stitching. The manufacturer can afford to spend more money on the details because he can charge more for the garment. All in all, good quality clothing is usually well worth the price.

Finding your own style is not easy. It takes patience and the willingness to experiment. It also involves an element of risk. Making an individual statement with your clothing implies making an individual statement about yourself. Yet, what many women are learning is that *no matter what you wear, you are saying something about yourself.*

Wear the best you can afford. Choose quality over quantity. Start with a basic Capsule and build around it. Let your personality show through. Every purchase you make for your wardrobe is an investment in your career. Let your clothes say who you are: an attractive, professional woman on your way to the top.